R.C. Reestad, PhD

Lung Function for the Clinician

Lung Function for the Clinician

D. T. D. Hughes M.A., B.Sc., B.M., B.Ch., F.R.C.P.
The London Hospital, Whitechapel, London E1

and

D. W. Empey M.B., B.S., M.R.C.S., M.R.C.P.
The London Chest Hospital, London E2

1981

ACADEMIC PRESS · London

GRUNE & STRATTON · New York

ACADEMIC PRESS INC. (LONDON) LTD
24-28 Oval Road,
London NW1

United States Edition published by
GRUNE & STRATTON
111 Fifth Avenue
New York, New York 10003

British Library Cataloguing in Publication Data

Hughes, D. T. D.
Lung function for the clinician.
1. Lungs–Diseases–Diagnosis
2. Pulmonary function tests
I. Title II. Empey, D. W.
616.2′4075 RC734.P84

Academic Press ISBN 0-12-792078-1

Grune & Stratton ISBN 0-8089-1369-7

LCCCN 81-80923

Printed in Great Britain by
St Edmundsbury Press, Bury St Edmunds, Suffolk

Preface

The object of this book is to present to clinicians those aspects of pulmonary function tests that are relevant to their practice. It attempts to explain the background of some of the tests commonly employed and how these may be useful in the clinical context. This involves some consideration of pulmonary physiology and a relatively superficial description of some of the lung function tests that are commonly employed. It is *not* a text book of physiology nor a technical manual of how to carry out the individual tests. Nor does it attempt to be comprehensive. There are other excellent publications that cover more comprehensively and in more detail the whole of clinical pulmonary physiology. These are listed at the end of Chapter Two. In contrast, this volume attempts to present something of a "bird's eye" view of the physiological background, and clinical interpretation and application of the more commonly employed tests. It is not aimed at the sophisticated pulmonary physiologist, but rather at the busy physician practising chest medicine. We hope it may prove useful, in fact, for a wider audience: for medical students, postgraduates in any field of Internal (General) medicine who seek guidance in interpreting results of lung function tests, and possibly for the increasing number of personnel such as technicians and others who are becoming involved in pulmonary function testing. Though it has a British "flavour" much of the material will be transportable across the water to North America, where both authors have worked and have clinical experience.

We wanted to produce a relatively simple, short monograph as opposed to a mini-textbook. For this reason a rather small number of references are cited. These are listed at the end of each chapter. Many refer to other excellent (but more detailed) works though some more specifically to particular methods or even to results in particular conditions. The Appendix contains a list of abbreviations and nomograms commonly used in predicting normal values.

January 1981

D.T.D.H.
D.W.E.

Contents

-1- Introduction

Specialised tests have the same importance in chest medicine as in all other branches of the science—they form part of the clinical approach which also involves history taking and physical examination. These tests may include chest radiography, blood tests, sputum examination, and lung function tests. In some cases, lung function tests are of prime importance in making a diagnosis, more usually they are a valuable adjunct in confirming a diagnosis, and sometimes they are indispensible as a way of monitoring the effect of treatment during certain respiratory illnesses.

Although Borelli first measured vital capacity in 1697, major advances in our understanding of pulmonary physiology have been made only in the past fifty years. The application of lung function tests to routine clinical medicine is an even more recent development, largely brought about by the introduction of portable, robust instruments. These need not be confined to the laboratory, but are also suitable for use in the surgery, and outpatients department. We hope that this book will help the non-specialist to obtain maximal information from the results of simple tests. The principles of the more important laboratory tests will be described and an indication will be given as to their usefulness and interpretation in particular diseases.

Application of lung function tests

The chief value of lung function tests lies in their use to detect abnormal *function*. They cannot indicate a precise anatomical or pathological diagnosis. Any disease present must, by its nature and extent be sufficiently severe to disturb the function of the lungs as a whole before most tests will detect any abnormality. It is also necessary that several types of test be performed so that patterns of abnormal function can be recognised. Thus, combinations of several tests may give much more information than a single test, and serial testing over a period may also yield far more information than studies carried out on one occasion only. Most of the tests employed were originally developed by physiologists and enable one to make a physiological rather than a pathological diagnosis. They will tell a doctor that the patient has airway obstruction, for example, but not that he has bronchial carcinoma. A number of situations in which lung function tests may be useful are listed below.

1. In differential diagnosis

A particular clinical picture or radiological appearance may be associated with more than one possible diagnosis. It may be that the lung function findings will help to decide the final diagnosis.

2. In objective assessment

This may be most important as it is not always easy to realise how severely a patient's lung function is impaired from his account of his symptoms. Actual measurements provide valuable objective evidence. They may be especially useful in assessing cases of *industrial lung disease* and the results of such tests are nowadays taken into consideration in deciding the amount of compensation due.

3. In determining the cause of dyspnoea

Lung function tests can often distinguish between pulmonary, cardiac and nervous causes of breathlessness.

4. In determining fitness for operation

This particularly applies to patients about to undergo thoracic operations when lung tissue will be removed. Pre-operative lung function tests may show the patient's likelihood or otherwise of surviving the resection of a lobe or lung without becoming a respiratory cripple.

5. As a guide to therapy

Here serial tests are of value. These may be done acutely—for example blood gas estimations done over a period of hours in a case of respiratory failure—or more chronically—for example serial estimations of the transfer factor over weeks or months in patients with sarcoidosis.

6. In drug trials

When a new bronchodilator drug is introduced, for example, its acute action in decreasing airway obstruction over a period of hours may be monitored and compared with that of a standard treatment and/or a placebo.

7. In asthma

Here the degree of airway obstruction varies from one day to the next and indeed from one time of day to another. Some asthmatics may be symptomless and have normal lung function measurements in the middle of the day when seen by the doctor, but may have much reduced measurements in the early morning and be severely dyspnoeic. If they are given a simple instrument such as a peak flow meter (see Chapter 3) and asked to make recordings throughout the day, the severity of their airway obstruction can be truly judged.

8. In neurological disease

Patients with poliomyelitis affecting the respiratory muscles are unable to breathe properly and often go into respiratory failure. This disease is uncommon now, but impaired lung function is found in some neuromuscular diseases such as myasthenia gravis and dystrophia myotonica. Lung function tests in these conditions can be informative.

9. In research

Measurements of pulmonary function may be used in disease research in two ways. They may define a particular pattern of deranged function in a particular disease, and may help us to understand in what way the physiology of patients with a particular disease is upset.

Thus there are a number of applications of lung function tests in clinical medicine. No *one* test is ideal. Some patients warrant intensive investigation as part of their initial assessment while, in others, it may be more valuable to make repeated simple measurements. The most information is often gained from a selection of tests. It is important that such tests are not carried out in isolation in the laboratory but that they are decided upon only after *clinical* appraisal of the patient. They may also need to be interpreted in the light of the patient's clinical condition. One should always remember, that the tests are relatively crude and that they are likely to give abnormal results only when diffuse disease is present to a relatively marked degree. We still have problems in the *early* detection of disease. Nevertheless, lung function tests are valuable in a number of clinical situations, many of which we hope to illustrate in the following chapters.

In this book, most of our attention is given to the simpler and more widely used tests of pulmonary function. However, some of the more complicated tests (e.g. compliance, exercise testing) are described briefly in Chapter 7. Each clinician and physiologist will have his own individual preference for particular tests and even for the methods by which particular measurements are made. References to a few general texts on pulmonary physiology are made at the end of this chapter, and more specific references are given at the end of other chapters as appropriate.

Conventional units have been used throughout with, where appropriate, the S.I. conversion factor given.

General references

Bates, D. V., Macklem, P. T. and Christie, R. V. (1971). *Respiratory Function in Disease.* 2nd Ed. London: W. B. Saunders.

Comroe, J. H. Jr. (1974). *Physiology of Respiration.* 2nd Ed. Chicago: Year Book Medical Publishers Inc.

Cotes, J. E. (1979). *Lung Function: Assessment and Application in Medicine.* 4th Ed. Oxford: Blackwell.

-2- Structure and function of the lungs

The principal function of the lungs is to facilitate gas exchange between the atmosphere and the blood. In carrying out this function, the lungs are involved in the respiration system which includes consumption of oxygen and production of carbon dioxide by the cells, transport of these gases between the tissues and the lungs by the blood, and gas exchange in the lungs. In this way, approximately 250 ml of oxygen are taken up from the atmosphere and 200 ml of carbon dioxide are excreted from the body every minute. The maintenance of a normal acid–base balance in the body also relies on normal lung function in that every day 20,000 mEq of hydrogen ions are excreted by the lungs as carbon dioxide compared with only 70 mEq excreted daily by the normal kidney. Before considering the clinical assessment of lung function and the changes which occur in disease, it is worth revising some of the essentials of lung structure and physiology (Cumming and Hunt, 1968).

General structure

The trachea branches into two main bronchi and these then subdivide into lobar bronchi, segmental bronchi, and so on for 27 generations (Fig. 2.1). The first 19 of these make up the conducting airways, which have no gas-exchange function; of these generations, the first seven are the cartilaginous airways or bronchi, while numbers 8–19 are membranous airways or non-respiratory bronchioles which end as terminal bronchioles. Generations 20–23 consist of respiratory bron-

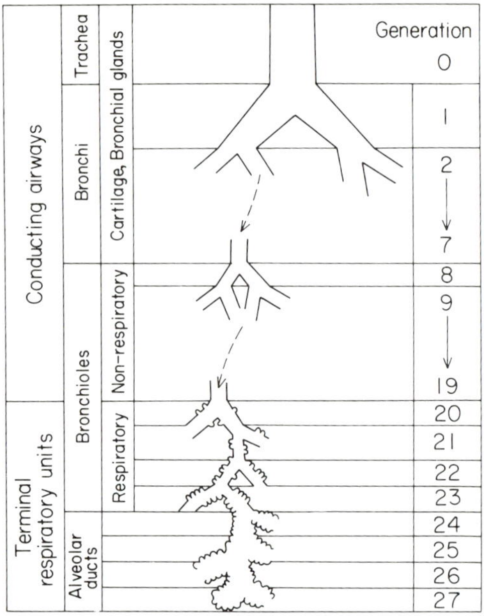

Fig. 2.1. *Schematic representation of the subdivisions of the conducting airways and terminal respiratory unit. Note that generation number begins with trachea (Adapted by Murray (1977) from Weibel (1963) and republished with permission of the publishers).*

chioles and 24–27 of alveolar ducts; both of these types of airway have alveoli arising from them and participate in gas exchange. The branches arising from a single terminal bronchiole are collectively known as the terminal respiratory unit. The conducting airways receive their blood supply from the bronchial arteries, which arise from the aorta and its branches. Together the cartilaginous bronchi and the non-respiratory bronchioles make up the bulk of the anatomical dead space, so called because air within it does not take part in gas exchange.

The cartilaginous airways decrease in size from the trachea and larger bronchi to bronchi of only about 2 mm in diameter. They are supported by incomplete rings of cartilage, and smooth muscle is also present. The non-respiratory bronchioles range from 2 mm to 0·6 mm in diameter. They lack cartilage and secretory glands but do have smooth muscle in their walls. In the larger bronchi, smooth-muscle contraction brings together tips of U-shaped cartilages. In the medium and small bronchi and bronchioles, because of the distribution of the muscle fibres in their walls, contraction reduces both the calibre and the length of the airways; thus producing increased rigidity as well as narrowing.

Terminal respiratory units

Distal to each terminal bronchiole are the airways from which the alveoli arise—these consist of respiratory bronchioles, alveolar ducts, atria, and alveolar sacs, which together are known as the terminal respiratory unit. The terminal respiratory unit is the site of gas exchange. The volume of gas within it is known as the alveolar volume and it is the ventilation of this region (alveolar ventilation) rather than the total pulmonary ventilation that determines the efficiency of gas exchange.

Some 25 million alveoli are present in man at birth, and these increase in size and number until there are more than 300 million in the healthy adult. The adult alveolar surface area is 80 m^2, 90% of which is covered with pulmonary capillaries; here the area of contact between the body and the external environment is 40 times greater than on the skin. The alveolar–capillary membrane is composed of the alveolar epithelium and its basement membrane, the capillary endothelium and its basement membrane, and the surfactant layer. Ninety-five per cent of the alveolar epithelial surface is made up of type I cells (squamous pneumocytes) which have broad cytoplasmic extensions only 0·1–0·3 mm thick. There are numerically more type II cells (granular pneumocytes) but they are cuboidal and occupy less than 5% of the alveolar surface. The type II cells have microvilli and contain lamellated inclusion bodies, which are believed to be associated with the production of surfactant. The capillary endothelium is formed by cytoplasmic extensions from endothelial cells. The alveolar epithelium and the capillary endothlium rest on separate basement membranes separated by an interstitial space containing elements of connective tissue. However, where the capillary bulges into the alveolus, the two basement membranes are fused. The capillaries meander in and out of the interstitial space, bulging into different alveoli as they go and forming a complex three-dimensional network.

Gas exchange takes place across the thin portion of the alveolar–capillary membrane where the basement membranes are fused. Diseases such as fibrosing alveolitis, which were previously thought to impair gas exchange by thickening this membrane ("alveolar–capillary block"), are now generally believed to create their major effects by destroying the balance between ventilation and perfusion. There is some evidence that the ultimate effect of airway obstruction on an individual patient may depend on the amount of collateral ventilation. The existence of the alveolar pores of Kohn, which allow gas to move between adjacent alveoli, and the canals of Lambert, which connect some respiratory and terminal bronchioles, is well recognised, but their functional importance–that is, how far they can compensate for airway obstruction–is not clear.

Lining the alveolar wall is a layer of surfactant, the principal component of which is dipalmitoyl lecithin. This lining film is crucial to normal respiration because it lowers the surface forces at the alveolar air–liquid interface, thereby reducing the work of breathing. As lung volume decreases, moreover, the presence of the surfactant reduces the surface tension even further and ensures the stability of the alveoli and peripheral airways. Increased stiffness of the lungs and multiple areas of pulmonary collapse are characteristic of diseases such as neonatal respiratory distress syndrome, in which the amount of surfactant is reduced.

Pulmonary vessels

The pulmonary arteries branch with the airways as far as the respiratory bronchioles and supply blood to the capillary network of the terminal respiratory units. The larger arteries are elastic and the smallest ones are muscular; autonomic innervation is from the sympathetic system. The pulmonary veins are thin-walled vessels which drain into the left atrium and have no fixed relation to the airways. The exact role of the supernumerary pulmonary arteries (not accompanying airways) and their corresponding veins remains to be defined. Although the output of the right ventricle equals that of the left, pulmonary artery pressure is much lower than systemic blood pressure. As the pulmonary circulation is a throughflow system, there is nothing analogous to the dead space of the airways.

The close structural relationship of the pulmonary arteries and airways means that any condition which impairs ventilation (such as collapse caused by a tumour) may also impair blood circulation to the relevant terminal respiratory units. This is advantageous since the optimal overall balance between ventilation and perfusion is maintained.

The pulmonary circulation also has non-respiratory roles. It filters blood to remove particles and emboli, and endothelial cells convert or break down such substances as angiotensin I and some of the prostaglandins.

Lymphatic vessels are found within the lung as the deep or parenchymatous lymphatic plexus, and on the surface as the pleural network. Most branches of the pleural network enter the lung, and lymph flows towards the hilum along the parenchymatous or interlobular channels. When enlarged in disease such as pulmonary oedema or lymphagitis carcinomatosa, the lymphatic vessels in the interlobular septa may appear on the chest radiograph as the familiar "Kerley B" lines.

Protective mechanisms

The larger airways are lined by ciliated, pseudostratified columnar epithelium, the thickness of which gradually decreases as the airways become smaller, so that the epithelium is only a single layer of almost cuboidal, ciliated cells in the terminal bronchioles. The cilia have a co-ordinated beating action (more than 1000 beats/min) that sweeps the mucus lining of the airways from the periphery towards the trachea and pharynx. The nose filters out most particles larger than 10 μm from the inspired air, and the multi-branching structure of the conducting airways encourages particles with aerodynamic diameters of between 2 and 10 μm to impact or settle on the airway surfaces. This serves to protect the alveoli from all but the very smallest particles. Particles that become trapped on the mucus lining of the airways are carried out of the healthy lung quite rapidly (less than 10 hours for 90% clearance), although there is wide individual variation in actual speeds of clearance. Coughing helps the clearance of larger collections of mucus. Soluble pollutants (such as sulphur dioxide) are removed by being dissolved in the fluid lining of the respiratory tract. Antibacterial substances and specific antibodies in the secretions of this tract play an important part in defending the lungs against damage.

The mucus layer is formed partly by goblet cells, which are found throughout the conducting airways; but the bulk of the secretions is produced by the bronchial glands. These are characteristic of the larger bronchi and are situated in the submucosal layer and connected to the surface by ducts. Irritants may cause discharge of the contents of the bronchial glands by a reflex mediated through the parasympathetic nervous system. Chronic irritation by cigarette smoke and other pollutants may contribute to chronic bronchitis, in which the bronchial glands increase in complexity and number of cells, and so produce more mucus.

Mast cells are found in the submucosa of the conducting airways. They resemble circulating basophilic leucocytes, but characteristic cytoplasmic granules can be shown by electron microscopy. The exact chemical content of human mast cells has not been determined but animal studies suggest that they contain histamine, proteolytic enzymes, and many other pharmacologically active substances. These are discharged in response to antigen–antibody reactions on the surface of the cell and thus may lead to asthma.

The alveoli are defended by alveolar macrophages. These phagocytic cells ingest any bacteria and other particles that reach the terminal respiratory units. Because of its probable importance in preventing many pulmonary infections, the alveolar macrophage is the subject of intensive research.

Innervation

The lung is innervated by branches of the vagus nerve and fibres from the upper four or five thoracic sympathetic ganglia. The airway smooth muscle is probably innervated both by parasympathetic and by sympathetic fibres, but physiological studies have shown that parasympathetic innervation predominates. The airway smooth muscle is, however, richly endowed with β-adrenergic receptors, which may respond to inhaled or circulating catecholamines causing smooth-muscle relaxation.

Within the airway epithelium, there are unmyelinated nerve endings, which are probably rapidly-adapting irritant receptors or "cough" receptors. These are mainly concentrated in the larger airways, and the afferent fibres travel in the vagus nerve. Such stimuli as irritant gases, pulmonary emboli, and pulmonary congestion may act on these irritant receptors to produce cough, hyperventilation, and bronchoconstriction. The non-specific bronchial hyper-reactivity that is so characteristic of asthma may be a manifestation of unduly sensitive irritant receptors, although the subject is controversial. Other receptors within the lung are pulmonary stretch receptors, which may affect breathing pattern in the newborn but which are probably not active after the neonatal period; and J receptors, which may contribute to the sensation of dyspnoea accompanying such diseases as pulmonary embolism and oedema.

Airway calibre and airflow resistance

As the bronchi and bronchioles branch within the lung, so their calibre decreases, but the total cross-sectional area of the airway increases with successive generations. Thus the velocity of airflow is reduced as air passes towards the periphery of the lung, and the bulk of the resistance to airflow is in the region with smallest cross-sectional area, i.e. the trachea and larger bronchi. As most of the simple lung function tests which attempt to detect changes in airway calibre are influenced by changes in airway resistance, they usually reflect changes in calibre of only the larger airways. The more peripheral airways (with a diameter of less than 2 mm) may be quite diseased and narrowed before any changes in airway resistance can be measured, and complex techniques are needed to show abnormal function in this "silent area" of the lung.

During inspiration the airways are distended, and during expiration their calibre is reduced. Airway narrowing may also be caused by mucosal swelling, mucus secretion, or contraction of the bronchial smooth muscle in response to chemical or nervous stimuli.

Basic clinical physiology

Lung function may be divided into four separate components, although these are closely inter-dependent. They are:

1. Ventilation—the mechanics of moving gases in and out of the lungs
2. Perfusion—the pulmonary circulation.
3. Gas exchange—the taking up of oxygen and the excretion of carbon dioxide.
4. Gas transport—the carriage of oxygen and carbon dioxide in the blood to and from the tissue.

Ventilation

Dead space

The normal adult breathes at a rate of approximately 15 times per minute inhaling roughly 500 ml of gas in each breath. This means that the minute volume of ventilation is 15 × 500 = 7500 ml/min. The conducting airways take no part in gas exchange, however, so their ventilation is wasted. They are referred to as the anatomical dead space. The volume of this dead space is proportional to body size, but an average value is around 150 ml for an adult. In addition, some alveoli (only at the apices in health but also elsewhere in disease states), may not receive any blood supply from the pulmonary circulation. These alveoli cannot take part in gas exchange and their ventilation is also "wasted". The volume of these alveoli forms part of the alveolar dead space. The rest of the alveolar dead space is accounted for by the ventilation of alveoli which have a *relatively* poor blood supply. These are being over ventilated relative to their needs for gas exchange, and the amount of this over ventilation can be quantified as the remainder of the alveolar dead space. The volume of the anatomical dead space and the alveolar dead space together is called the physiological dead space. In health this is almost the same as the anatomical dead space, say 150 ml in an adult, but in disease states it may be as large as 350 ml. Even if the dead space is normal in size, the volume of gas actually entering the alveoli with each breath is only 500 − 150 = 350 ml. The minute ventilation of the alveoli will thus be 15 × 350 = 5250 ml/min. It is the gas involved in this alveolar ventilation which is actually taking part in gas exchange and which is of utmost importance.

A fall in tidal volume will reduce alveolar ventilation even if the total minute volume of ventilation is kept the same. A second example will illustrate this. If tidal volume = 250 ml and respiratory rate = 30 breaths/min, minute volume of ventilation = 7500 ml/min as before. But alveolar ventilation = (250 − 150) × 30 = 3000 ml/min. This is much lower than the 5250 ml/min in the earlier example.

An increase in the physiological dead space will have a similar effect in reducing alveolar ventilation if tidal volume is kept the same. Normally the physiological dead space is 35% or less of the tidal volume, but it may rise to 60 or 70% of the tidal volume in some diseases. It is important to realise that one cannot deduce alveolar ventilation simply by measuring the minute ventilation at the mouth, and that it is alveolar ventilation which is of prime importance. The best method of assessing the adequacy of alveolar ventilation is to measure the arterial $P\text{CO}_2$ (see Chapter 5).

Lung volumes

The lungs are normally closely applied to the chest wall—separated from it by only a thin layer of fluid—the pressure in the pleural space being a few centimetres of water below atmospheric pressure. If the chest is opened, the lungs deflate. This is caused by the elastic recoil which results from stretched elastic fibres and surface tension forces within the alveoli. The chest wall has an inherent springiness and the ribs tend to spring outwards. When a subject is fully relaxed, i.e. not using any respiratory muscles, as occurs at the end of a normal gentle expiration, the elastic recoil of the lung inwards is exactly balanced by the tendency of the ribs to spring outwards. This position of equilibrium is the end expiratory point and the volume of the lungs at this point is called the functional residual capacity (FRC). The normal pattern of breathing is to commence at the FRC by contracting the external intercostal muscles which swing the ribs upwards and outwards, and by contracting the diaphragm downwards. This increases the volume of the thorax and lowers and intra-thoracic pressure, so that the lungs are expanded. If there is an increased resistance to air flow, the accessory muscles of respiration such as the sternomastoids may have to be used. Expiration normally involves no active muscular effort; the muscles of inspiration are relaxed and the lungs and chest wall return to their position of equilibrium (FRC). In conditions such as chronic bronchitis, asthma or emphysema the resistance to air flow is greater during expiration, and it may be necessary to use the muscles of expiration even in quiet (tidal) breathing. These are the internal intercostal muscles, which swing the ribs downwards and inwards, and the abdominal muscles which raise the intra-abdominal pressure and push the diaphragm upwards. Diseases such as myasthenia gravis or dystrophia myotonica which affect the muscles of respiration or those such as poliomyelitis which affect the nerves supplying them, can obviously have serious effects on lung function.

If the deepest possible breath is taken in and the lungs are expanded to their largest possible volume, this volume is called the total lung capacity (TLC). If a maximal expiration is now performed, until no more gas can be exhaled, the volume of gas expired is called the vital capacity (VC). Inevitably some gas must remain in the lungs as the chest wall does not completely collapse when we breathe out. This remaining volume is called the residual volume (RV). It is clear that VC + RV = TLC. The factors determining these and the other lung volumes and capacities in health and disease are discussed in Chapter 4, together with methods of measuring them.

The conducting airways

Air initially enters the nasal passages and pharynx and then passes into the trachea and the branching bronchial tree. The structure of this system has already been described above. Flow in the largest airways is fast and turbulent, but in the smaller airways it is slower and more laminar in nature. Flow has virtually ceased by the time the respiratory bronchioles are reached, and simple diffusion is responsible for the movement of gases in and out of the alveoli themselves.

Difficulty in inflating the lungs may occur because the lungs are stiff, or because there is a rigid chest wall, or it may be the result of an increased resistance to the flow of air through the airways. Airway obstruction may be partial or complete and may be caused by the presence of a foreign body, blockage with mucus, swelling of the lining mucosal surface of the bronchi or contraction of the airway smooth muscle. The physiological effects of airway obstruction are discussed in Chapter 8.

Compliance of the lungs

If the lungs are abnormally stiff they will be harder to inflate. In this case, the compliance of the lungs is said to be reduced. Methods of measuring compliance and the clinical significance of changes in compliance are discussed in Chapter 7.

The work of breathing

The respiratory muscles perform work in stretching the elastic tissues of the lung, in moving the chest wall, and in overcoming frictional resistance to air flow in the airway. In the normal subject, the amount of work performed is not large, the oxygen used being only 1–3% of the total oxygen consumption of the body. In patients with stiff lungs or with an increased frictional resistance to airflow, the work of breathing may be greatly increased, particularly during exercise. When the lungs are abnormal, an altered pattern of breathing may result in the greatest economy with regard to oxygen consumption. An increase in airway resistance will lengthen the time which the lungs will take to fill for any given degree of effort; this means that slow, deep breaths will ventilate the lungs with the greatest efficiency. Conversely, a fall in compliance will mean that rapid shallow breathing will produce the greatest ventilation with the minimum of effort. In this case, the dead space will still be ventilated and so the total ventilation will have to be increased if the same alveolar ventilation is to be achieved.

Many diseases alter airway resistance, compliance and physiological dead space, and so the actual pattern of breathing which will be optimal for any one patient is difficult to predict.

Control of ventilation

The respiratory centre controls the rate and depth of breathing. It is in the medulla and produces a rhythmic discharge of nerve impulses which results in a regular breathing pattern. The respiratory centre is sensitive in normal people to changes in carbon dioxide tension ($P\text{CO}_2$) in the arterial blood. Deviation of the arterial $P\text{CO}_2$ away from fairly narrow limits results in appropriate adjustment of the pattern of breathing. In addition to this mechanism, there are chemoreceptors in the aorta and carotid body which respond to hypoxia and reflexly stimulate respiration. This mechanism is less important in normal people, but in a patient with chronic bronchitis whose respiratory centre has diminished responsiveness to changes in $P\text{CO}_2$, this reflex is the chief drive for respiration (see Chapter 5).

Perfusion

The structure and function of the pulmonary circulation has already been described. Blood flow through the lungs does, of course, depend on adequate cardiac function. In addition, gravity affects the circulation markedly because of the low pressures involved.

With a mean systolic pressure of only 25 mm Hg it is easy to see that when we are standing, the apices of our lungs may only just be perfused or may not be perfused at all by pulmonary arterial blood. Another factor affecting pulmonary blood flow is hypoxia which will cause widespread pulmonary arterial vasoconstriction. Of greatest importance in clinical medicine, however, is the way in which ventilation and perfusion are matched together, a failure of this matching being the major cause of the hypoxaemia seen in many lung diseases. We shall give only a brief outline of this concept here. A book by John West, listed at the end of the chapter, is recommended to those with a particular interest in this subject.

Matching of perfusion and ventilation

The pulmonary capillary perfusion matches the alveolar ventilation on roughly a one to one basis. For example, 5000 ml of blood pass through the capillaries every minute and 5250 ml of air per minute ventilate the alveoli. This balance of ventilation and perfusion is crucial if efficient gas exchange is to take place, and it is usually expressed in a shorthand manner. Alveolar ventilation is written as $\dot{V}_A$, the V meaning the volume of gas and the dot indicating that it is measured over a period of time. The suffix A means that the volume is alveolar gas. The pulmonary capillary perfusion is written as $\dot{Q}$, the Q meaning volume of blood, and the dot again meaning that it is measured over a period of time. We can now say that the $\dot{V}_A/\dot{Q}$ ratio for the lungs is 5250/5000 which is approximately equal to one. This would seem to be ideal, but it is only the overall $\dot{V}_A/\dot{Q}$ ratio and takes no account of regional variations in the lungs. If, for example, all the ventilation of 5250 ml/min was of the alveoli in the left lung where as all the perfusion of 5000 ml/min was in the right lung, although the overall $\dot{V}_A/\dot{Q}$ ratio was still approximately equal to 1·0, gas exchange would be impossible. The alveoli in the left lung would have a $\dot{V}_A/\dot{Q}$ ratio of $5250/0 = \infty$ and those in the right lung would have a ratio of $0/5000 = 0$. These are clearly the two extremes. In practice the majority of the alveoli have $\dot{V}_A/\dot{Q}$ ratios of between 0 and ∞, and most of them in health have values near to 1·0.

Effects of abnormal $\dot{V}_A/\dot{Q}$ on gas exchange

Figure 2.2 shows three alveoli. The middle one has the ideal $\dot{V}_A/\dot{Q}$ ratio of 1·0 whereas that on the left has a ratio of ∞ and that on the

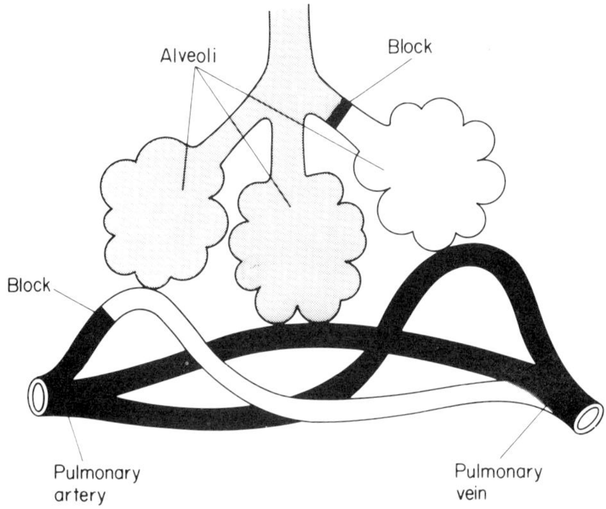

Fig. 2.2. *Diagramatic representation of ventilation and perfusion to three hypothetical alveoli (see text for explanation).*

right one of 0. The alveolus which has ventilation but no perfusion ($\dot{V}_A/\dot{Q} = \infty$) is part of the alveolar dead space. As such, its ventilation is wasted and it forms part of the physiological dead space. Any alveolus with a $\dot{V}_A/\dot{Q}$ ratio $> 1{\cdot}0$ will be receiving relatively more ventilation than it needs to match its perfusion, and the higher the ratio, the greater the amount of wasted ventilation. Thus, for those alveoli with high $\dot{V}_A/\dot{Q}$ ratios, a proportion of their ventilation is effectively part of the physiological dead space. This is referred to as the dead space effect. Clinical situations in which there may be alveoli with high $\dot{V}_A/\dot{Q}$ ratios are pulmonary embolism and pulmonary hypertension. The effect of these conditions on gas exchange is the same as that of making the dead space larger.

Similarly, an alveolus with perfusion but no ventilation ($\dot{V}_A/\dot{Q} = 0$) will not take part in gas exchange. Its perfusion is wasted, and the blood from it has the same content of gases as the mixed venous blood from the right side of the heart. The effect of this is the same as if there were a direct pulmonary artery to pulmonary vein anastomosis (or a shunt from the right to the left side of the heart) and it is called the venous admixture effect. Any alveoli with $\dot{V}_A/\dot{Q}$ ratios <1 will have some perfusion which is greater than appropriate to their ventilation. The amount of this wasted perfusion is said to contribute to the venous admixture effect. Clinical conditions in which this may occur are pulmonary oedema, in which fluid in the alveoli prevent ventilation but blood flow may continue, and consolidation or collapse of the lung, when ventilation of parts of the lung is reduced or absent.

Local adjustment of ventilation/perfusion ratios
Although several examples have been taken to illustrate the principles of $\dot{V}_A/\dot{Q}$ mis-matching, it must be pointed out that there are mechanisms for some local regulation of ventilation and perfusion. If an airway is partially or completely occluded, the diminished or absent ventilation of the alveoli it serves will lead to local hypoxia. This will cause pulmonary artery vasoconstriction in the area concerned, and the $\dot{V}_A/\dot{Q}$ ratio will become more normal as perfusion is reduced. Similarly, occlusion of the pulmonary artery supplying particular alveoli leads to loss of surfactant in those alveoli, and hence to a reduction in their compliance and therefore in their ventilation. This again will tend to adjust the $\dot{V}_A/\dot{Q}$ ratio towards normal.

Gas exchange

The structure of the lungs is such that blood is brought into very close contact with the inspired air. The factors controlling the exchange of gases between the alveoli and the capillary blood in the lungs are explained in Chapter 5.

Gas transport

Oxygen is carried in the blood, mainly in combination with haemoglobin. Carbon dioxide is carried as either bicarbonate, in simple solution, or combined with proteins as carbamino compounds. Further details are given in Chapter 5.

References

Cumming, G., Hunt, L. B. (Editors). (1968). *Form and Function in the Human Lung*. Edinburgh: Livingstone.
Murray, J. (1977). *The Normal Lung*. London: W. B. Saunders.
Weibel, E. R. (1963). *Morphometry of the Human Lung*. Berlin: Springer Verlag.
West, J. B. (1970). *Ventilation/Bloodflow and Gas Exchange*. 2nd Ed. Oxford: Blackwell.

Part of this chapter is reproduced, with permission, from Empey, D. W. (1978). Structure and function of the lungs. *British Medical Journal* **1**, 631–633.

-3- Ventilatory function

Assessment by simple tests

The ability of a patient to move gas in and out of the lungs is described as his ventilatory function. Impairment of this function is one of the commonest problems in chest disease. The simplest method of assessing ventilatory function is to use a spirometer (Fig. 3.1) to record the volumes of gas inhaled and exhaled on a revolving drum. In this way a graph of volume against time is obtained (Fig. 3.2). The spirometer can be used to measure several volumes and capacities, the most important of which is the *vital capacity* (VC). This is the volume of gas which can be exhaled after a maximal inspiration. Inevitably this is not equivalent to the total amount of gas in the lungs, as the lungs cannot be completely emptied. The remaining gas is called the *residual volume* (RV) and this together with the vital capacity makes up the *total lung capacity* (TLC). The spirometer alone cannot measure RV or TLC (see Chapter 4).

If the recording drum is moving at a known speed, and the subject is asked to exhale with maximal effort after a deep inspiration, a trace similar to that shown in Fig. 3.2 is obtained. The vital capacity recorded is known as the *forced vital capacity* (FVC) in this case as maximal effort was used during expiration. The time is marked so that the total time taken for expiration and the amount of gas expired after one second can be measured. Normal subjects should expire their whole vital capacity in less than three seconds and about three-quarters of it in one second. The second of these measurements, known as the *forced expired volume in one second* (FEV_1), is a very useful test for airway obstruction.

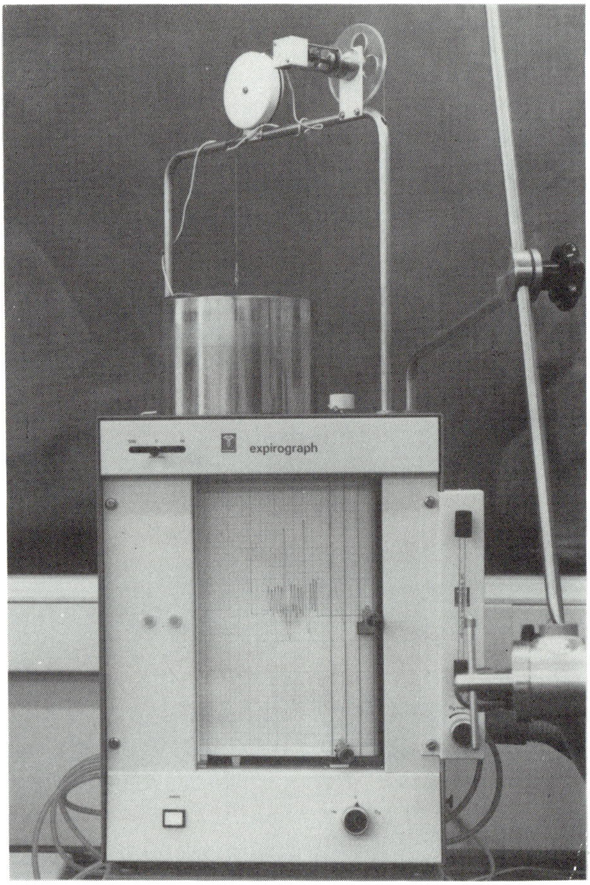

Fig. 3.1. *Expirograph water-sealed spirometer.*

Various types of spirometer are available (see Wever, Britton and Hughes, 1976). The water-sealed bell spirometer offers a low resistance and inertia and is theoretically the most satisfactory model (Fig. 3.1). There are many minor modifications of this spirometer type available. It is cumbersome, however, and in clinical practice a dry spirometer of the type shown in Fig. 3.3 is more useful (Drew and Hughes, 1969). This kind of spirometer records (Fig. 3.4) only the expiratory phase of the spirometer tracing shown in Fig. 3.2. Pressure sensitive paper avoids the use of an inked pen, and the "bellows" construction avoids the need for water seals. The patient is instructed to take a deep breath in, place the mouthpiece between the lips and

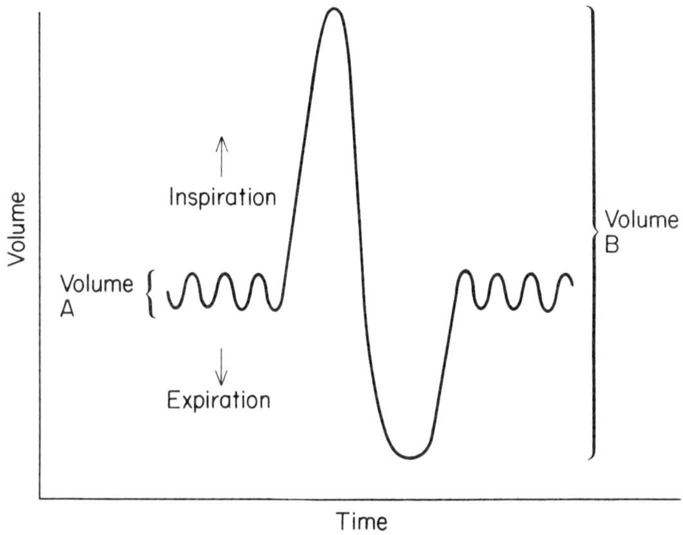

Fig. 3.2. *Trace obtained from the expirograph spirometer. Volume A = quiet or "tidal" breathing i.e. tidal volume. Volume B = vital capacity; the volume of gas which can be exhaled after the deepest possible inspiration.*

then exhale steadily until no more gas can be expelled. This is the so called static measurement of the vital capacity. Several recordings of forced expiration are now made and the FVC and FEV_1 are measured. In normal subjects the static VC and the FVC do not differ significantly, but in some conditions, the high intrathoracic pressures generated by forced expiration cause premature closure of the airways with trapping of air in the chest. This occurs in emphysema and makes the FVC markedly lower than the static VC. All of these measurements, recorded with either type of spirometer, are made at ambient temperature and pressure (ATP) but should be corrected to allow for body temperature and pressure and saturation with water vapour (BTPS) representing the conditions inside the lungs. This can be done by a simple multiplication of the volume by a correction factor (see Appendix 4 for details).

The VC, and hence the FEV_1, will vary in volume according to a variety of factors such as the age, sex and height of the subject. It is greater in men than in women, decreases with age and is proportional to the height of the subject. Numerous measurements of VC have been made in many different populations and it is now possible

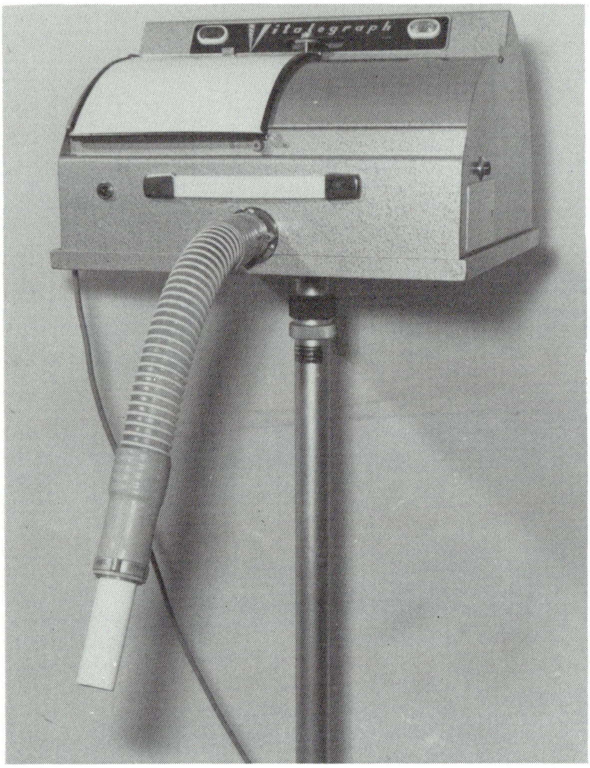

Fig. 3.3. *Vitalograph dry spirometer*

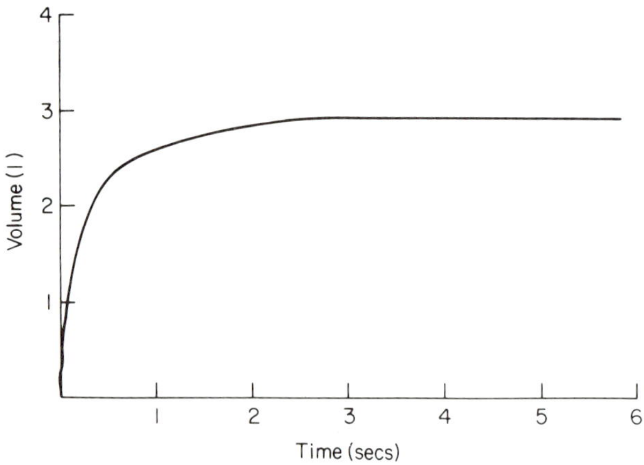

Fig. 3.4. *Expiratory trace obtained from the Vitalograph spirometer.*

to predict the value expected for any individual (see Appendix 2). Even so, there are wide variations and a value of between 75% and 125% of the predicted value should be accepted as normal. The FEV_1 can be similarly predicted. The proportion of the VC which is represented by the FEV_1 is expressed as the FEV% which is (FEV_1/FVC) × 100%. This is normally 75% but the value falls with increasing age and may even be as low as 55% in normal elderly persons.

Another approach in assessing ventilatory function is to measure *flow rates*. These can be recorded from spirometer traces, the rate being calculated after drawing a tangent to the curve. This method is not very accurate, however. The best method is to use a pneumotachograph (see Chapter 7), but these are not always avail-

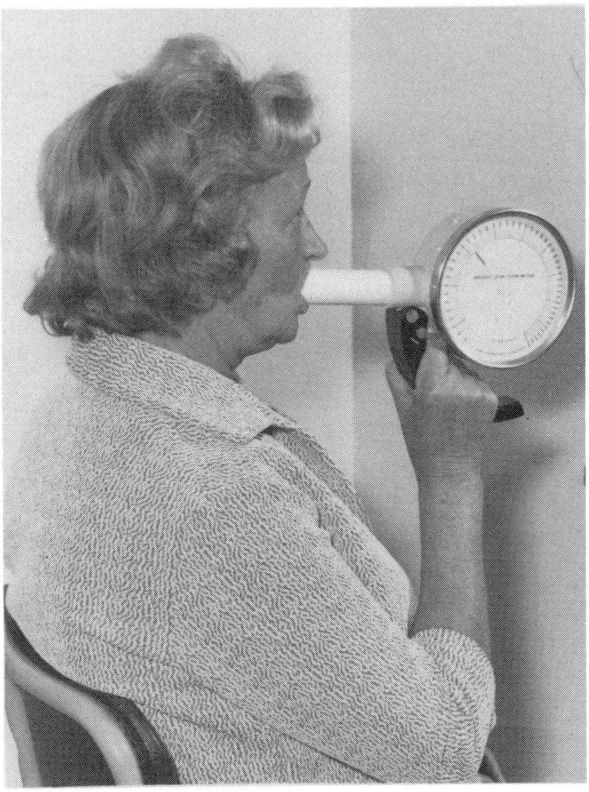

Fig. 3.5. *Wright peak flow meter in use (reproduced by permission of the Editor, Hunterian Society Transactions).*

able. A useful compromise is the Wright peak flow meter (Fig. 3.5). This instrument is portable and gives helpful results when used in conjunction with a spirometer or, in some situations, alone. The instrument contains a vane which is displaced during forced expiration after a maximal inspiration. The degree of displacement is proportional to the flow rate which is recorded on a dial. The reading on the dial is the greatest flow rate which is maintained for at least 10 milliseconds. This means that a cough will not produce a misleadingly high reading as the resulting high flow rates are sustained for less than 10 milliseconds. Predicted values can be obtained from nomograms for *peak expiratory flow rate* (PEFR). In general most men should be able to achieve more than 400 l/min and women more than 300 l/min.

Changes in disease

These simple tests of ventilatory function can be used to distinguish two different patterns of disease from each other and from the normal. These are the so-called obstructive and restrictive patterns, and are best illustrated by clinical examples as described below and in Fig. 3.6.

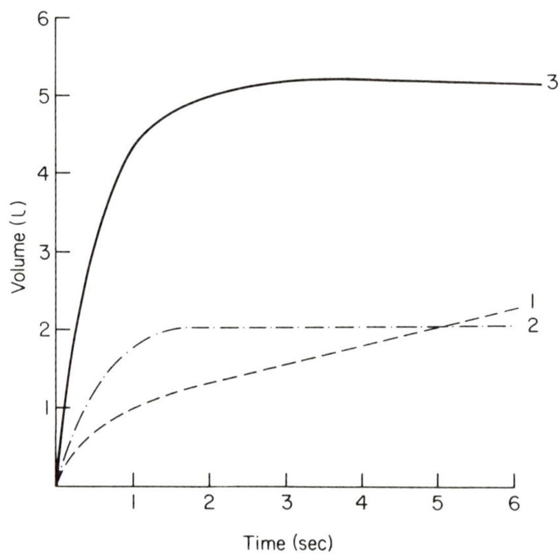

Fig. 3.6. *Vitalograph spirometer traces from: 1. Patient with airway obstruction; 2. Patient with restrictive defect; 3. Normal subject.*

Example 1

Mr J. E. is 65 years old, smokes heavily and complains of chronic cough and breathlessness.

	Actual	*Predicted*	*% Predicted*
FVC (ml)	2300	3950	58
FEV_1 (ml)	1000	2800	36
FEV%	43%	71%	
PEFR (l/min)	155	520	30

The FVC is reduced, but the most marked changes are the reductions in FEV_1, FEV% and PEFR. The fact that only half of the FVC can be exhaled in one second and the actual reductions in FEV_1 and PEFR to 36% and 30% of predicted normal respectively, points to obstruction of the airways in this case. The diagnosis was chronic bronchitis and the results are typical of the obstructive pattern.

Example 2

Mrs. M. J. is 40 years old and has had increasing breathlessness without cough for several years.

	Actual	*Predicted*	*% Predicted*
FVC (ml)	2000	3100	65
FEV_1 (ml)	1750	2600	67
FEV%	88%	84%	
PEFR (l/min)	420	400	105

In this case the FVC is reduced but the FEV_1 is only reduced proportionately. The FEV% is still normal as is the peak expiratory flow rate. There is, therefore, no airways obstruction but there is a reduction of the vital capacity. The diagnosis was found to be fibrosing alveolitis and these results are typical of the restrictive pattern of disease. The causes of this pattern are listed in Chapter 9.

Example 3

Mr B. C. is a healthy 22-year-old student.

	Actual	*Predicted*	*% Predicted*
FVC (ml)	5200	5000	104
FEV_1 (ml)	4300	4200	102

FEV%	83%	84%	
PEFR (l/min)	600	625	96

These results are entirely normal.

Use of bronchodilators

In cases where airway obstruction has been demonstrated, it is useful to know whether or not this is reversible. Isoprenaline, a bronchodilator, can be given by means of an aerosol spray, and the tests repeated after 10 minutes. An improvement of more than 15% may be taken to demonstrate significant reversibility of the airway obstruction.

Example 4
Mrs K. M. is 30 years old and has allergic asthma.

	Actual	*Predicted*	*% Predicted*	*After isoprenaline*	*% Change*
FVC (ml)	2100	3300	64	2450	+17
FEV_1 (ml)	1250	2800	45	1650	+32
FEV%	60%	85%		67%	
PEFR (l/min)	170	430	40	220	+29

The obstructive type of pattern (reduced FEV_1, FEV% and PEFR) is shown with significant improvement in FVC, FEV_1 and PEFR after isoprenaline. The FEV_1 has improved by a greater percentage than the FVC, and this has led to a rise in FEV%. While this indicates an improvement in the airway obstruction, the FEV% should never be considered alone when assessing this condition (see Chapter 8). The large improvements in FEV_1 and PEFR seen in this case are typical of asthma. N.B. Failure to respond to a single dose of isoprenaline does not exclude asthma—more intensive therapy may be needed to demonstrate reversibility.

Large airway obstruction

It may be obvious that a patient has developed an obstruction of the trachea or larynx if, for example, a large goitre is present and there is loud inspiratory stridor. In some cases, however, the diagnosis is not suspected clinically, and the stridor may even be mistaken for wheeze arising from within the chest. In such circumstances, the first pointer towards the correct diagnosis may come from observation of the spirometer trace and the peak flow readings obtained in the pulmonary function laboratory.

Example 5
Mrs J. E. is 43 years old with a long history of recurrent laryngeal stenosis.

	Actual	*Predicted*	*% Predicted*
FVC (ml)	2600	3200	81
FEV_1 (ml)	1300	2600	50
FEV%	50%	81%	
PEFR (l/min)	70	400	18

FEV_1/PEFR ratio = 18.6

$P\text{CO}_2$ = 56 mmHg

In this example, the FVC is normal and there is moderate reduction in the FEV_1 and the FEV%. The PEFR, however, is greatly reduced and the $P\text{CO}_2$ is elevated, indicating respiratory failure.

Close inspection of the spirometer tracing (Fig. 3.7) shows that the

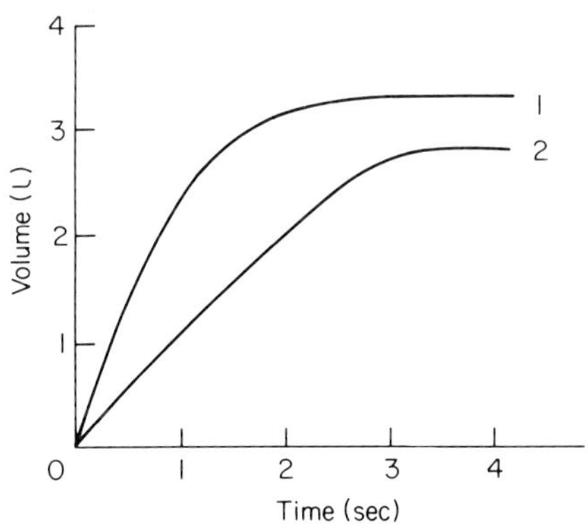

Fig. 3.7. *Vitalograph spirometer traces from: 1. Normal subject; 2. Subject with large airway obstruction.*

line is virtually straight as compared to the curve which is normally seen. This is a characteristic of large airway obstruction and together with a disproportionately low PEFR as compared to the other indices, should alert the clinician to this possibility. A numerical value of the relationship between the PEFR and the FEV_1 can be obtained by dividing FEV_1 expressed in mililitres by PEFR expressed in litres per minute. The resulting number (which is in arbitrary units) is usually less than 10.0 in normal subjects, subjects with restrictive lung disease, and subjects with asthma, chronic bronchitis, or emphysema. If significant large airway obstruction is present, this ratio usually exceeds 10 and higher values usually indicate more severe degrees of obstruction (Empey, 1972).

It must be emphasised that if large airway obstruction is suspected clinically, a normal FEV_1/PEFR ratio does not exclude it and further studies including flow volume curves (see Chapter 7) and endoscopy are indicated. The only value of this ratio lies in alerting the clinician to the possible presence of a hitherto unsuspected lesion.

Additional measurements of flow rates

Forced mid-expiratory flow (FMF)

Although the usual flow rate measured is the peak expiratory flow rate (PEFR), it is possible to measure rates of flow at different times during a forced expiratory manoeuvre or to measure the average rate of flow over certain periods during the manoeuvre (Fig. 3.8).

The average flow rate over the middle part of the forced vital capacity is now called the forced mid-expiratory flow (FMF)—it was previously known as the maximum mid-expiratory flow rate. Sometimes this measurement is referred to as the $FEF_{25\text{–}27\%}$ i.e. the average forced expiratory flow as the middle 50% of the vital capacity is exhaled.

The instantaneous flow rates at various points on the spirogram can also be measured. It is, however, more usual to read these off a flow volume curve (see Chapter 7). Examples of instantaneous flow rates include $FEF_{50\%}$, which is the expiratory flow rate when 50% of the vital capacity has been exhaled, and $FEF_{75\%}$, which refers to the point when 75% of the vital capacity has been exhaled.

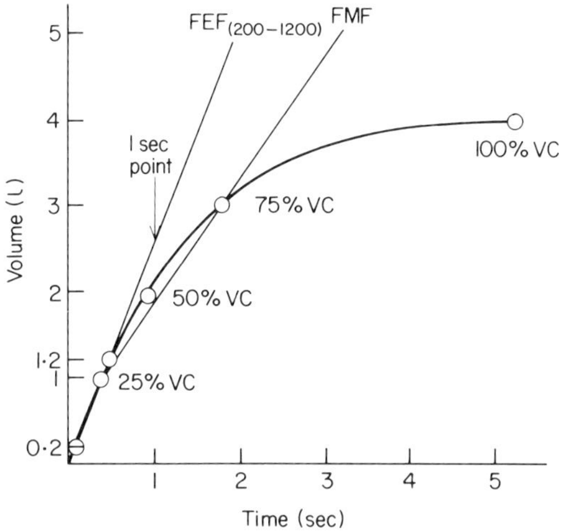

Fig. 3.8. *Expiratory spirogram showing derivation of* $FEF_{(200-1200)}$ *and FMF. To measure FEF join points on spirogram representing volumes of 0·2 and 1·2 litres on volume scale. Extend this line. The volume achieved in one second on this extended line is the FEF in l/sec (just under 3 l/sec in this example). For FMF join points on curve corresponding to volumes at 25% and 75% of VC (namely one and three litres in this example. Continue line and derive FMF from its slope—i.e. measure volume in one second along this straight line (about 1·3 l/sec in this example).*

Some laboratories measure the average rate of flow for the expiration of one litre of gas commencing 200 ml after the start of a forced expiration. This is known as the $FEF_{200-1200}$ and was originally introduced as a strategy for discarding the initial portion of the spirogram which was sometimes variable.

In clinical practice, these sub-divisions of the spirogram or flow volume curve are not always necessary and for most purposes measurement of the FEV_1, PEFR and VC is sufficient. Many authorities use the FEV_1 as a numerical value, but look at the actual traces of the expiratory spirogram whenever possible. Similarly the *shape* of the flow volume curve (Chapter 7) may be as, or even more, useful than the $FEF_{50\%}$ value derived from it.

Maximum voluntary ventilation (MVV)

Maximum voluntary ventilation (MVV)—alternatively known as maximum breathing capacity (MBC)—is another measurement that

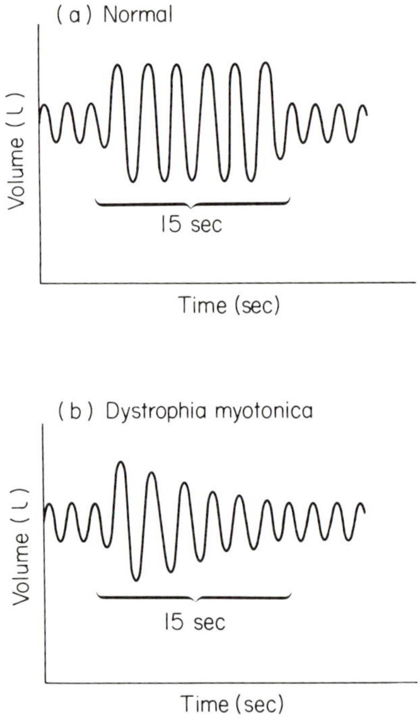

Fig. 3.9. *(a) Normal maximum voluntary ventilation (MVV) trace from water-sealed spirometer. (b) Trace in patient with dystrophia myotonica. Note the effect of muscle fatigue which causes the amount of ventilation to decrease.*

has rather gone out of fashion. To measure it, a subject was asked to breathe as deeply and quickly as possible for 15 seconds into a water filled spirometer and a trace similar to that shown in Fig. 3.9a was obtained. This ventilation over a 15 second period was multiplied by four to give a MVV value in litres per minute. Although the MVV was reduced in airways obstruction, the trace reflected not only the degree of airways obstruction but also the actual power and efficiency of the respiratory muscles. In patients with muscle disease, it would look like that shown in Fig. 3.9b. Patients with severe airways obstruction would become very dyspnoeic and distressed during the performance of the test. For this reason an indirect index was developed. After theoretical consideration, it was felt that multiplying the FEV_1 by 37.5 would give a maximum breathing capacity (indirect MBC) similar to that obtained by direct measurement. This is true in normal subjects and may be true in some patients with chest disease, although it is certainly not true in patients with muscle weakness. For example, in dystrophia myotonica the indirect MBC is greater than the direct value since the muscles become easily fatigued (Lee and Hughes, 1964). There is thus no real advantage in using an indirect MBC instead of an FEV_1 in chest disease.

References

Drew, C. D. M. and Hughes, D. T. D. (1969). Characteristics of the Vitalograph spirometer. *Thorax* **24**, 703–706.

Empey, D. W. (1972). Assessment of upper airways obstruction. *Br. Med. J.* **3**, 503–505.

Lee, F. I. and Hughes, D. T. D. (1964). Systemic effects in dystrophia myotonica. *Brain* **87**, 521–524.

Wever, A. M. J., Britton, M. G. and Hughes, D. T. D. (1976). Evaluation of two spirometers: A comparatives study of the Stead–Wells and the Vitalograph spirometers. *Chest* **70**, 244–520.

-4- Lung volumes

The *vital capacity* (VC) is the maximum volume of gas that can be expelled from the lungs by forceful effort following maximal inspiration. If this is expired into a spirometer of some sort, the volume can be measured. This is not the *total* lung volume, however, since all of the air contained in the lungs cannot be expelled during life however great an effort is made. There are various reasons for this which include:

1. The structure of the lungs themselves. The spongy nature of the alveoli and the relatively rigid and non-collapsible structures such as the trachea and bronchi.

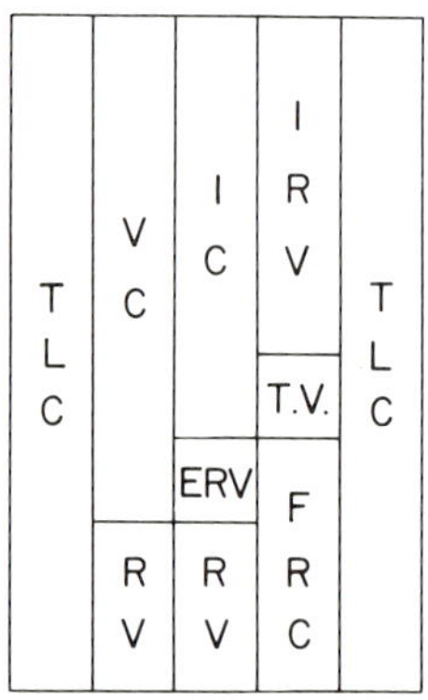

Fig. 4.1. *Diagram showing lung volumes. TLC = Total lung capacity, VC = vital capacity, RV = residual volume, IRV = Inspiratory reserve volume, TV = Tidal volume, FRC = Functional residual capacity, ERV = Expiratory reserve volume, IC = Inspiratory capacity.*

2. The negative intrathoracic pressure which transmits the outward pull of the thoracic cage to the lung.
3. The presence of pulmonary surfactant which prevents alveolar collapse at low lung volumes and thus their complete emptying of air.

Methods have been evolved to measure the "non-expellable" gas in the lungs and hence the total lung size. These were developed along three main lines, described below. The terms used in these descriptions were originally standardised by a group of American physiologists over 20 years ago (Pappenheimer, 1950) and are shown diagrammatically in Fig. 4.1.

Methods used to measure lung volumes

Closed-circuit helium dilution method

The insoluble, inert gas helium is used so that none will leave the alveolar gas to enter the bloodstream. A water-sealed spirometer system of known volume (V_{App}) is filled with a mixture of helium and air (about 10% helium). This is the initial helium concentration or He_I. The patient is then connected to the system (Fig. 4.2) and continues to breathe the helium mixture until the helium concentration in the circuit falls to a constant level. The final level (or He_F) has been produced by the dilution of the original helium caused by the additional volume of the subject's lungs. A vital capacity manoeuvre is made when the helium concentration is apparently stable, and values for vital capacity (VC) and for expiratory reserve volume (ERV) are read off the spirograph trace. This manoeuvre also ensures that all parts of the lung are open to enable a complete degree of helium dilution to occur. If He_F drops further, this implies that air (not containing helium) has been released from parts of the lung not in communication with the helium mixture during the quiet tidal breathing. If need be, the vital capacity manoeuvre is repeated several times until the helium concentration *is* constant. We know the initial and final helium concentrations and the volume of the apparatus. Since no helium enters or leaves this closed system, it is possible to calculate the unknown lung volume as shown:

$$V_{App}He_I + V_L He_L = He_F(V_{App} + V_L)$$
$$V_{App}He_I + 0 = He_F V_{App} + He_F V_L$$

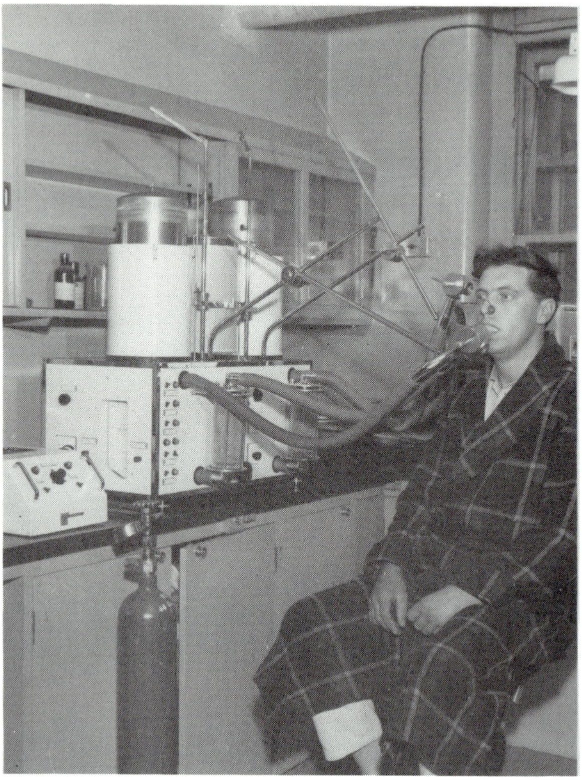

Fig. 4.2. *Measurement of lung volumes by the closed circuit helium dilution method.*

$$\mathrm{He}_F V_L = \mathrm{He}_I V_{App} - \mathrm{He}_F V_{App}$$

$$V_L = \frac{V_{App}(\mathrm{He}_I - \mathrm{He}_F)}{\mathrm{He}_F}$$

where V_L = Unknown lung volume (in this case FRC) to be measured

V_{App} = Volume of spirometer system

He_L = Helium concentration in lung at start = 0

He_I = Initial helium concentration in system

He_F = Final helium concentration in system.

As the subject is connected to the spirometer system at the end of expiration of a tidal breath, this volume is therefore the patient's functional residual capacity. To obtain the residual volume (RV), the expiratory reserve volume (ERV) must be subtracted, since RV = FRC–ERV.

Helium concentration is estimated using a katharometer, an instrument which responds to the thermal conductivity of the gas. The instrument is accurate but has a relatively slow response time. Normal subjects reach a constant helium concentration in about 2 minutes. Patients with airways obstruction, particularly those with emphysema, may take 10 minutes or more to reach equilibrium and will also need several vital capacity manoeuvres. Even then a true equilibrium may not have been reached since some intrathoracic gas may be trapped behind occluded airways or in bullae and never come into contact with the helium mixture. This volume of non-ventilated intrathoracic gas can be measured by the plethysmographic method, described in this Chapter.

Nitrogen washout method

This depends on the following principle as illustrated in Fig. 4.3. There is an *unknown* volume of gas (in this case FRC) in the subject's lungs. The nitrogen (N_2) content of air *is* known, however (about 80%). If the *amount* of nitrogen in the lungs could be estimated, the total volume of alveolar gas could be calculated. The amount of nitrogen in the lungs is determined by "washing it out" and measuring its concentration. This is done by making the patient breathe nitrogen-free oxygen and then collecting the expired air in a spirometer previously flushed out with pure oxygen. The subject breathes pure oxygen for 7 minutes and the expired gas is collected in a spirometer so that its volume and nitrogen concentration can be determined. The calculations are then as follows:–

Volume of expired gas collected in spirometer $= V_S$

Concentration of nitrogen in this case $= F\mathrm{N}_2$

Amount of nitrogen collected in spirometer $= V_S \times F\mathrm{N}_2$

$= V\mathrm{N}_2$

But $V\mathrm{N}_2$ was originally present in the lungs as 80% N_2

∴ Total alveolar volume $= V\mathrm{N}_2 \times 100/80$

In practice, small corrections must be made for any nitrogen removed from the body's stores when the partial pressure of nitrogen was

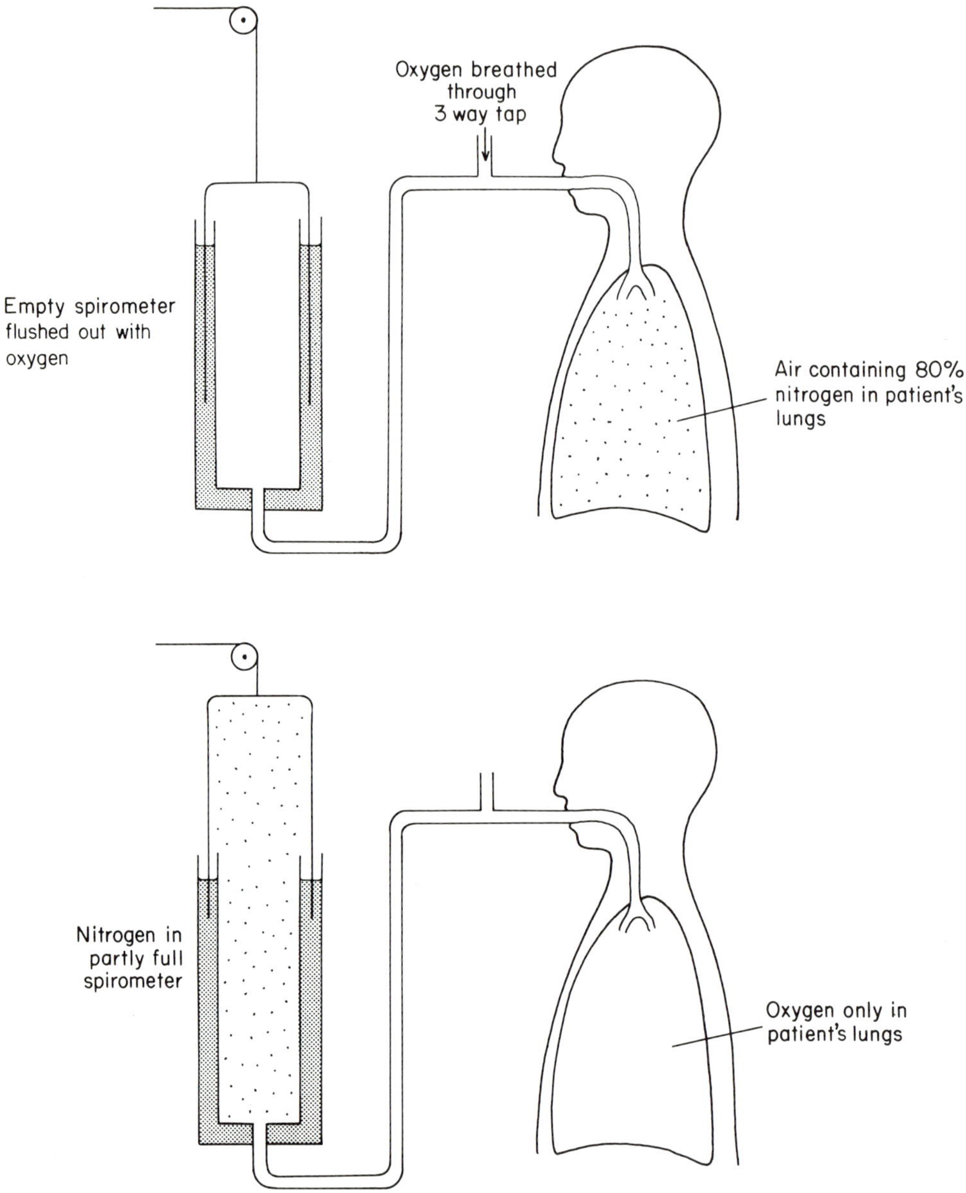

Fig. 4.3. *At the start of the experiment, the patient's lungs are filled with air containing approximately 80% nitrogen. He then breathes pure oxygen* in *through the 3 way valve and breathes* out *into the large spirometer. At the end of the experiment, his lungs contain virtually pure oxygen whilst the spirometer contains most of the nitrogen from his lungs.*

lowered by breathing oxygen; also for any traces of nitrogen contained in so-called 100% oxygen. As in the previous method, there may be "non-ventilated" areas, the nitrogen of which is not available to contribute to the estimation.

Body plethysmographic method

It is possible to use the constant volume body plethysmograph to measure the total volume of gas in the thorax whether this is in communication with the airways or not. This is termed the thoracic gas volume (TGV). In normal subjects this volume will be similar to the FRC measured by either of the methods already described. In diseases such as emphysema, however, it may exceed the FRC by as much as a litre or more. This measurement of the TGV is based on Boyle's law which states that the product of the volume (V) and pressure (P) of a given gas in a closed system remains constant provided that the temperature does not change. Thus if the volume changes, the pressure will also change i.e. $PV = P'V'$. The subject sits in the body box with the airtight door closed and quietly breathes air through a mouthpiece. At end-expiration the mouthpiece is occluded by an electrically controlled shutter whilst the patient continues to breathe against this obstruction. The effects of this manoeuvre are as follows: at end-expiration, alveolar pressure = atmospheric pressure = P and V is the unknown thoracic gas volume. An attempted inspiration against the occluded shutter enlarges the thorax and so decompresses the intrathoracic gas; this in turn creates a new thoracic gas volume V'; also a new pressure P' which is measured by the gauge in the airway between the patient's mouth and the occlusion. Since there is no flow of gas, mouth pressure is assumed to equal alveolar pressure. The increase in the thoracic gas volume (ΔV) is estimated from the rise in box pressure detected by the very sensitive pressure transducer. We have therefore now measured P, P' and ΔV and can determine V as follows:

$$\begin{aligned} PV &= P'V' \\ &= P'(V + \Delta V) \\ &= P'V + P'\Delta V \\ \therefore PV - P'V &= P'\Delta V \end{aligned}$$

$$\therefore V(P - P') = P'\Delta V$$

$$\therefore V = \frac{P'\Delta V}{P - P'}$$

This method is rapid and simple. The only drawbacks are the expense and complexity of the apparatus (illustrated in Fig. 4.4) and the requirement of a skilled technician or doctor to operate it. For these reasons, use of the body box tends to be confined to larger medical centres. The method is well described by Dubois *et al*. (1956). A good comparison of the three different methods described above has also been made (Tierney and Nadel 1962).

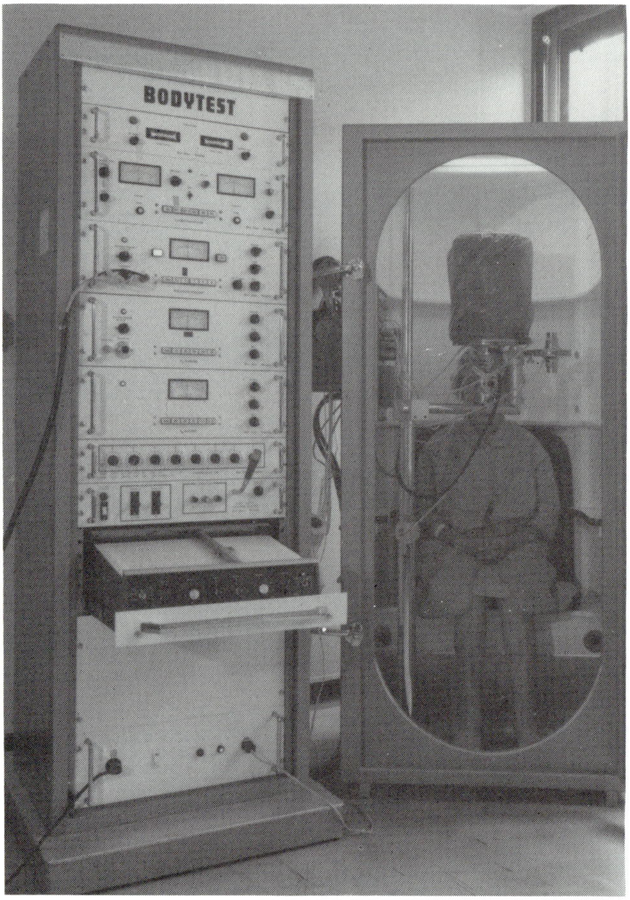

Fig. 4.4. *Body plethysmograph.*

Value of lung volume measurements

Measurements of lung volumes are really "static" rather than "dynamic" and do not represent the changing pattern during respiration. Nevertheless they can be valuable in clinical practice since a number of diseases affect them. Furthermore the measurement of lung volumes is a relatively simple procedure which is easily performed. A number of quite large series of normal subjects have had their lung volumes measured and prediction formulae have been produced. Most of these are of the form $VC = F_1 \times H - F_2 \times A \pm K$ where F_1 and F_2 are factors, H is the height and A the age of the subject and K a constant (see Appendix 2). The several formulae so far produced agree remarkably well. Thus it is possible not only to measure a patient's actual vital capacity, but to compare it with what it should be. Normally, the residual volume should be only a quarter of the total lung capacity i.e. RV/TLC = 0·25. This ratio increases with age, but even so, it is safe to state that for subjects up to 60 years old, the RV/TLC ratio should not normally exceed 0.4. In cases of severe airways obstruction, particularly in emphysema, the actual RV may be increased to 200% of the predicted value or more, and this ratio may be as high as 0·7. This represents gross hyperinflation of the lungs with air trapping. In some cases of early emphysema, the VC may be relatively well preserved so that the actual TLC is greater than 100% of predicted. Most lung diseases, however, tend to produce a *fall* in VC and other lung volumes. In restrictive lung disease (such as fibrosing alveolitis or kyphoscoliosis), all the lung volumes are reduced proportionally so that the RV/TLC ratio remains normal. As emphysema progresses or in bronchitis, the VC is reduced. Even so the FVC (made as a forced expiration with no time limit) is never reduced as much as the FEV_1 in which a one second time limit is applied (See Chapter 3).

It is of value to record the patient's pattern of tidal breathing while lung volume is being measured by the helium dilution or nitrogen washout method. Most normal subjects will breathe evenly (Fig. 4.5) although they may tend to hyperventilate (in a regular pattern) due to the somewhat artificial situation of being connected to a mouthpiece and a system of definite resistance. Patients with anxiety or compensation neurosis often produce a characteristic irregular breathing pattern (Fig. 4.6).

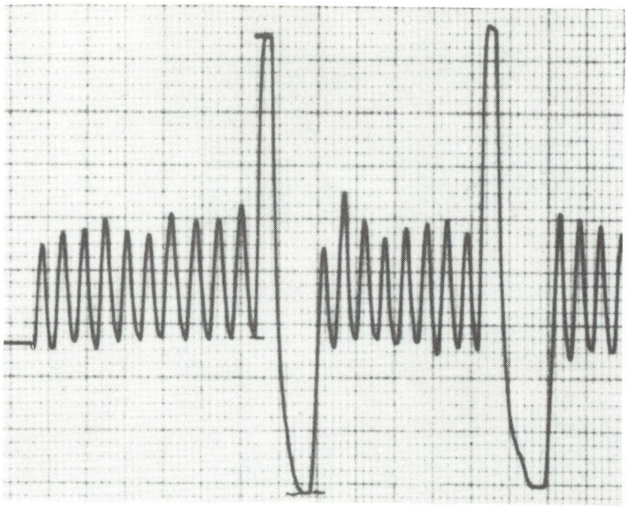

Fig. 4.5. *Spirographic trace showing breathing pattern in normal subject.*

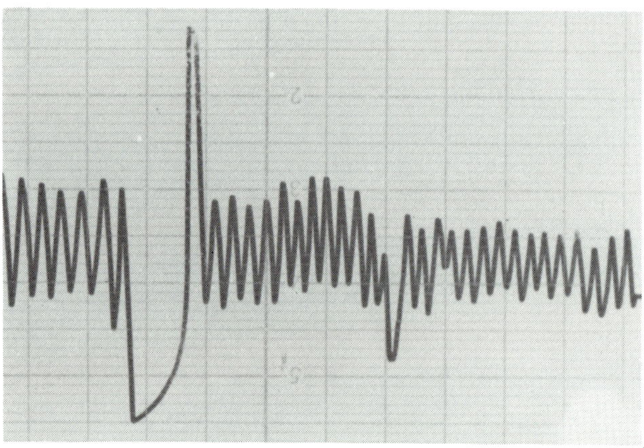

Fig. 4.6. *Spirographic trace showing irregular breathing pattern in anxious subject.*

References

Dubois, A. B., Botelho, S. Y., Bedell, G. N., Marshall, R. and Comroe, J. H. (1956). A rapid plethysmographic method for measuring thoracic gas volume. *J. clin. Invest.* **35**, 322–326.

Pappenheimer, J. (1950). Standardisation of definitions of symbols in respiratory physiology. *Fedn. Proc.* *9*, 602–605.

Tierney, D. F. and Nadel, J. A. (1962). Concurrent measurements of functional residual capacity by three methods. *J. Appl. Physiol.* **17**, 871–873.

-5- Gas exchange

We have already mentioned that the main purpose of the lungs is to achieve exchange of gases between the alveoli and the bloodstream. The net effect of this is that carbon dioxide is excreted from the body and oxygen is taken up by the blood. For this exchange to take place efficiently, several conditions must be satisfied. Firstly, the lungs must be sufficiently large. If the surface area of alveoli has been reduced by the destruction of alveolar walls in emphysema or by surgical resection of the lung, there may not be a large enough surface area of alveolar membrane in contact with the pulmonary capillaries for sufficient gas exchange to occur. Secondly, the alveolar ventilation must be adequate to replenish the oxygen in the alveoli and to wash out the carbon dioxide. Similarly, the pulmonary circulation must be intact to supply the alveolar capillaries with blood. As well as being sufficient in quantity, ventilation and perfusion must be to the same alveoli as explained in Chapter 2. That is to say that for gas exchange to be at its most efficient, the $\dot{V}_A/\dot{Q}$ ratio must be approximately equal to one.

Gas partial pressures

In any mixture of gases, the pressure exerted by any one gas (i.e. its partial pressure) is equal to the total pressure multiplied by the fraction of the total amount of gas which it represents. The notation for partial pressure is a capital italic P and a suffix is usually added to denote whether this is the partial pressure of inspired gas (P_I) or the partial pressure of alveolar gas (P_A) or the partial pressure of gas in arterial blood (P_a). If a mixture of gases is in contact with and equilibrated with a liquid, each gas in the mixture is dissolved in the liquid to an extent determined by its partial pressure and its solubility in the liquid. The partial pressure of a gas in a liquid is that pressure at which it would produce the concentration of gas molecules found in the liquid if it were in the gaseous phase in equilibrium with the liquid.

The composition of dry air is approximately 21% oxygen, 78% nitrogen and 1% inert gases and carbon dioxide. The barometric pressure at sea level is 760 mmHg and so the partial pressure of oxygen in dry air (PO_2) is $0{\cdot}21 \times 760 = 160$ mmHg.* Similarly, the PN_2 is $0{\cdot}78 \times 760 = 593$ mmHg. Usually, however, there is some water vapour in the air which reduces these values and, when air reaches the lungs, it is fully saturated with water vapour. The PH_2O at body temperature when the air is fully saturated is 47 mmHg. Thus the PO_2 of air entering the lungs is $(760 - 47) \times 0{\cdot}21 = 150$ mmHg (P_IO_2). This air mixes with the dead space gas and the gas already in the alveoli. As oxygen is entering the blood from the alveoli, and carbon dioxide is being liberated, the composition of alveolar gas is

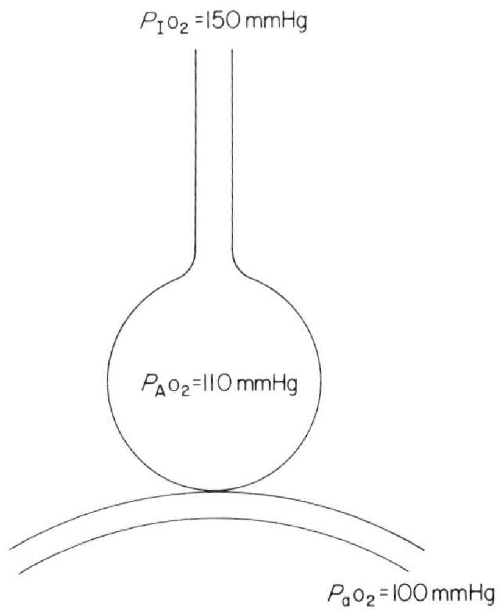

Fig. 5.1. *Oxygen gradient between inspired air and pulmonary capillary blood.*

*See Appendix 1 for conversion to SI units.

such that the P_AO_2 is lower than that of the inspired gas and the P_ACO_2 is higher. This is shown in Figure 5.1. The partial pressure of oxygen in the arterial blood leaving the lungs (P_aO_2) is shown as 10 mmHg lower than the P_AO_2. This is normal because of the small amount of "shunt" which occurs in the lungs. If the right to left shunt effect is large, however, with blood by-passing the alveoli which are being ventilated then the alveolar–arterial oxygen tension gradient ($P_AO_2 - P_aO_2$) will be greater than 20 mmHg. The usual PO_2 in mixed venous blood arriving at the lungs ($P_{\bar{v}}O_2$) is 40 or 50 mmHg. This is approximately 60 mmHg lower than the alveolar PO_2. The $P_{\bar{v}}CO_2$ is normally 46 mmHg and is thus 6 mmHg higher than the normal P_ACO_2.

It should now be easy to appreciate that from the moment when oxygen is taken in at the mouth to the time when it reaches the mitochondria in the tissues, it is passing from areas of higher partial pressure of oxygen to areas of lower partial pressure of oxygen.

Exchange of gases

The alveolar gas is separated from the blood by a very thin partition. This consists of the alveolar lining cell membranes the interstitial fluid, the capillary lining cell membranes, the plasma and the red cell membranes (Fig. 5.2). The overall thickness of this barrier is one or two μm and it offers only minimal resistance to the diffusion of gases across it. Both oxygen and carbon dioxide diffuse passively across this barrier at rates dependant on their solubility and on differences in their partial pressure on either side. Although the partial pressure difference for carbon dioxide is only 6 mmHg, it is much more soluble than oxygen and diffuses with ease. The partial pressure difference for oxygen is approximately 60 mmHg which is also sufficient to allow passive diffusion to take place.

At rest, nearly all the oxygen diffusion takes place in one-third of the time during which the blood is in the pulmonary capillary. Even during exercise, there is time for the process to be completed. It used to be thought that the hypoxia that occurred in such diseases as pulmonary fibrosis was due to a diffusion block for oxygen caused by thickening of the alveolar walls. It has been shown in recent years that these conditions produce sufficient changes in compliance to disturb

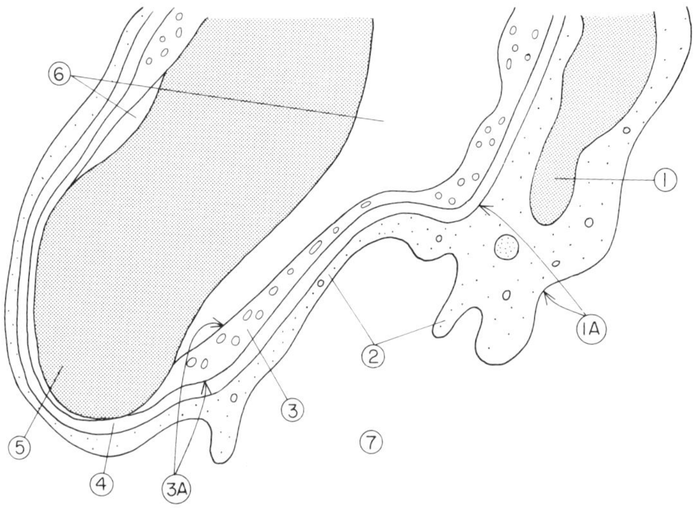

Fig. 5.2. *Diagram of electron micrograph of pulmonary alveolar–capillary membrane. 1. Nucleus of alveolar cell; 1A. Alveolar cell lining membranes; 2. Cytoplasm of alveolar cell; 3. Cytoplasm of pulmonary capillary endothelium; 3A. Capillary lining cell membranes; 4. Interstitial fluid; 5. Red blood cell within capillary; 6. Plasma in lumen of pulmonary capillary; 7. Alveolar space.*

the ventilation/perfusion relationship and that it is this which explains the hypoxia seen in these conditions. In practice, the efficiency of gas exchange can be determined by measuring the transfer factor (see Chapter 6).

The uptake of oxygen by the blood depends on chemical reactions in the red blood cells where oxygen combines with haemoglobin molecules in stages until the haemoglobin is fully saturated with it. The amount of oxygen which can be taken up depends on the rate of chemical reaction between the haemoglobin and the oxygen, and on the amount of haemoglobin present in the blood. Carbon dioxide is carried mainly as bicarbonate in the plasma. In the lungs this diffuses into the red cells and there combines with hydrogen ions to form H_2CO_3. This is then dehydrated by carbonic anhydrase to form H_2O and CO_2. The CO_2 then diffuses back into the plasma and across the alveolar–capillary membrane into the alveoli.

Gas transport in the blood

Oxygen

Oxygen is chiefly carried in combination with haemoglobin. The small amount which is in solution in the plasma is not significant at normal atmospheric pressures. One gram of haemoglobin can carry 1·39 ml of oxygen and thus, one litre of blood, with the normal haemoglobin concentration of 14 g/l can carry 19·6 ml of oxygen. The degree of saturation of the haemoglobin varies with the partial pressure of oxygen in the blood. The familiar S-shaped dissociation curve (Fig. 5.3a) illustrates this. Haemoglobin is 95% saturated at a PO_2 of 90–100 mmHg and it is still 90% saturated when the PO_2 is 60 mmHg. Below this level of PO_2 however, the degree of saturation of the haemoglobin rapidly falls and a lot of oxygen is given off for very small changes in PO_2. One result of this curve is that over-ventilation of parts of the lung cannot make up for under-ventilation elsewhere. This is because any increase in PO_2 above 90 or 95 mmHg will cause only a minute rise in the volume of oxygen actually taken up by the blood.

Carbon dioxide

Carbon dioxide is carried in the blood in three main ways—as bicarbonate, which accounts for the majority; in simple solution, and combined with proteins as carbamino compounds. Carbon dioxide diffuses from the tissues into the red blood cells where the enzyme carbonic anhydrase catalyses the reaction $CO_2 + H_2O = H_2CO_3$ forming carbonic acid. This dissociates into hydrogen ions and bicarbonate, the released hydrogen ions being buffered by the haemoglobin in the red cell. The reverse process occurs in the lungs. The dissociation curve for carbon dioxide is shown in Figure 5.3b. The key difference between the dissociation curves of carbon dioxide and oxygen is the steepness of the CO_2 curve throughout its length. This means that much greater volumes of carbon dioxide are given off for small changes in partial pressure compared with oxygen. Over-ventilation of some parts of the lung resulting in a lower PCO_2 will thus increase diffusion, compensating for low diffusion rates in any part of the lung

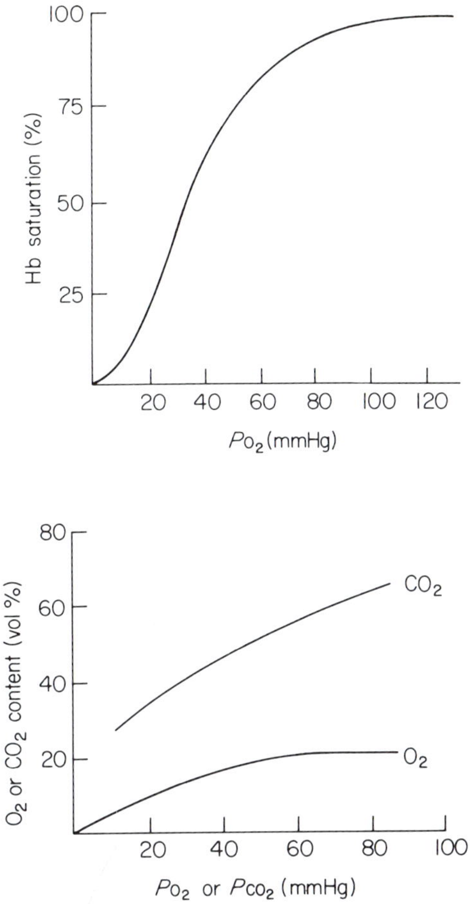

Fig. 5.3. *(a) Oxygen dissociation curve for haemoglobin. (b) Dissociation curves for carbon dioxide and oxygen in blood.*

which is under-ventilated. This is markedly different from the situation with oxygen where no such compensation can occur.

Blood gas tensions

In Chapter 2 we briefly considered the significance of blood gas tensions in health. We must now consider the effects of disease and treatment (Donald *et al.*, 1952). The "ideal" alveolar gas composition

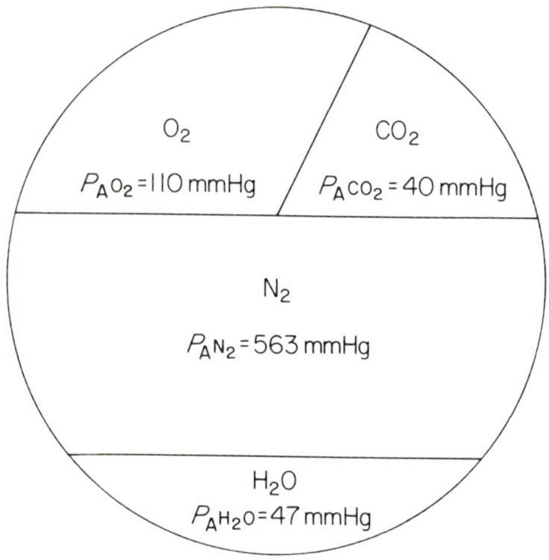

Fig. 5.4. *Usual composition of alveolar gas.*

in health is diagramatically shown in Figure 5.4. The gas is saturated with water vapour and at 37°C so the P_AH_2O is 47 mmHg and constant. The normal, healthy subject would be breathing air and so the P_AN_2 is constant at 563 mmHg. The P_AO_2 and P_ACO_2 are the only variables, and there is a linear relationship between them. Clearly when breathing air P_AO_2 and P_ACO_2 must add up to 150 mmHg i.e. the P_IO_2 gas tension. As one increases, the other decreases and vice versa. This is shown in Figure 5.5. The slope of the line is dependant on R

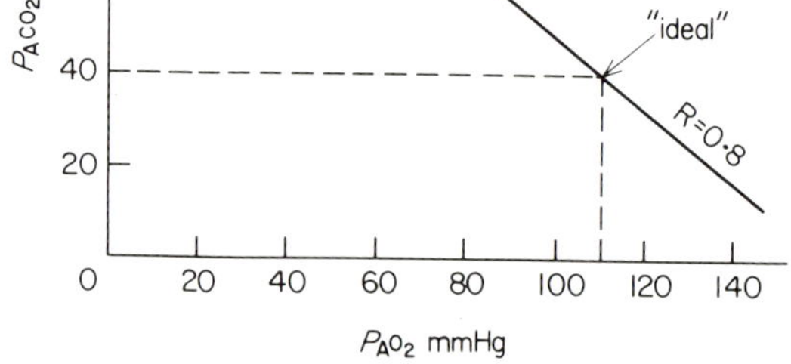

Fig. 5.5. *Relationship between alveolar* P_{CO_2} *and* P_{O_2}.

(the respiratory exchange ratio, i.e. carbon dioxide elimination divided by oxygen uptake), and the "ideal" alveolar air point is shown. The elimination of carbon dioxide depends on the alveolar ventilation (see below) such that if the subject hypoventilates while the metabolic rate remains unchanged, the P_ACO_2 will rise. Inevitably, the P_AO_2 will fall simultaneously. This is shown in Figure 5.5. If one measures arterial blood gases, the P_aCO_2 will roughly equal P_ACO_2, while the P_aO_2 will be lower than the P_AO_2, although by not more than 20 mmHg in health.

Respiratory failure

Respiratory failure can best be defined by reference to blood gas tensions. The strict limits for normal blood gas tensions are P_aCO_2 35–45 mmHg and P_aO_2 80–100 mmHg. Respiratory failure is defined as a rise in the P_aCO_2 above 50 mmHg or a fall in the P_aO_2 below 60 mmHg. In some conditions, however, such as pulmonary fibrosis, the P_aO_2 may fall below 60 mmHg while the P_aCO_2 is also lowered or remains normal. These conditions are usually referred to as causing respiratory insufficiency rather than respiratory failure. The term respiratory failure is commonly reserved in clinical practice for those conditions in which the P_aCO_2 rises above 50 mmHg.

The patient with chronic obstructive bronchitis may go into respiratory failure at an early stage of the disease. When he suffers an acute exacerbation, his P_aCO_2 may be as high as 70 or 75 mmHg on admission to hospital. It is well known that the chronic bronchitis patient in respiratory failure has lost his responsiveness to carbon dioxide as a drive to ventilation. Instead his chronic hypoxia drives the respiratory centre. Administering oxygen in any amount may increase the P_aO_2 sufficiently to diminish the drive to ventilation and thus allow the P_aCO_2 to rise even higher. The higher the concentration of oxygen given, the more likely this will be to happen. To make matters worse, the administration of oxygen also allows the P_aCO_2 to rise to much higher levels than it could when breathing air. This is because the added inspired oxygen washes out nitrogen until a new alveolar gas composition is achieved. The P_ACO_2 can now rise to much higher levels for any given P_AO_2. This is shown diagramatically in Figure 5.6, and some actual values are shown in Table 5.1.

The patient in respiratory failure with a P_ACO_2 of 90 mmHg will

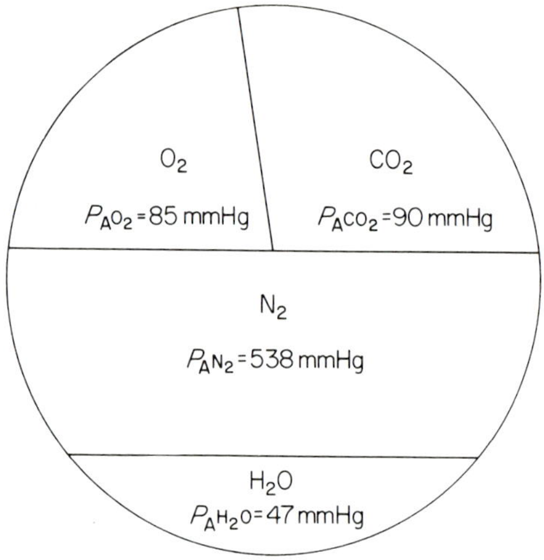

Fig. 5.6. *Alveolar gas composition in hypoventilating patient breathing air with increased oxygen content.*

have a P_AO_2 of 60 mmHg in the "ideal" alveolus. If the P_IO_2 is increased from 150 mmHg (air) to 175 mmHg (24% oxygen) the range of P_AO_2 and P_ACO_2 will be as shown in Table 5.1. The increased P_IO_2 may cause a rise in P_aO_2 and hypoventilation can occur. The P_AO_2 will then fall to 60 mmHg again, but with the reduced alveolar ventilation, the P_ACO_2 will rise to 115 mmHg. Similarly, the effect of using 28% oxygen (P_IO_2 = 200 mmHg) will be to cause the P_AO_2 to remain at 60 mmHg. Clearly a P_ACO_2 of 140 mmHg could never occur

Table 5.1. *Effect on alveolar gas composition in respiratory failure (mmHg) of breathing air containing different concentrations of oxygen*

	21% O_2 (normal air)	24% O_2		28% O_2	
		Worst	Best	Worst	Best
P_AO_2	60	60	85	60	110
P_ACO_2	90	115	90	140	90
P_AN_2	563	538	538	513	513
P_AH_2O	47	47	47	47	47
Total	760	760	760	760	760

when breathing air—the P_AO_2 could then only be 10 mmHg and this would be quite incompatible with life. If hypoventilation does not occur, but the P_ACO_2 is kept at 90 mmHg, the P_AO_2 will of course rise as shown in the "Best" column in the Table. If the P_ACO_2 can rise to 140 mmHg when only 28% oxygen is being used, it is clear that higher concentrations of oxygen can be potentially even more dangerous in susceptible patients.

Oxygen therapy in practice

From the preceding paragraph it will be clear that oxygen is potentially a dangerous drug and that as such it should only be prescribed by a doctor who is well aware of the side effects and consequences. It is necessary to identify those patients who are at risk so that appropriate concentrations of oxygen can be given from the beginning. The patients most at risk are those who are already in respiratory failure with a high P_aCO_2 and those in borderline respiratory failure. These patients will have diminished responsiveness of the respiratory centre to carbon dioxide. The situation is worse with these patients if they have received sedative drugs of any type. The patient at risk may be known from previous admissions to be in chronic respiratory failure. Patients who have the typical clinical history of chronic bronchitis will also be suspected of possibly being in respiratory failure even if there are no previous measurements of arterial carbon dioxide available. Although there are some clinical features of carbon dioxide retention (drowsiness, confusion, bounding pulse and warm peripheries, coarse tremor etc.) it is usually impossible to estimate P_aCO_2 by any means other than by measurement. The techniques for this are discussed below.

The decision to administer oxygen is based on recognition of arterial hypoxaemia which is considered severe enough to be harmful to the patient. In general, there is little point in administering oxygen to patients whose arterial PO_2 is above 40 or 45 mmHg. The clinical diagnosis by estimating the degree of cyanosis may be misleading because of the presence of polycythaemia in many of these patients. Blood gas tension measurements should be made initially and, if the P_aO_2 is low enough, oxygen therapy should commence. If the P_aCO_2 is elevated above 50 mmHg initially, therapy should be given using a mask which delivers 24% oxygen. These masks (Fig. 5.7) are usually based on the Venturi principle. The small increase in P_IO_2

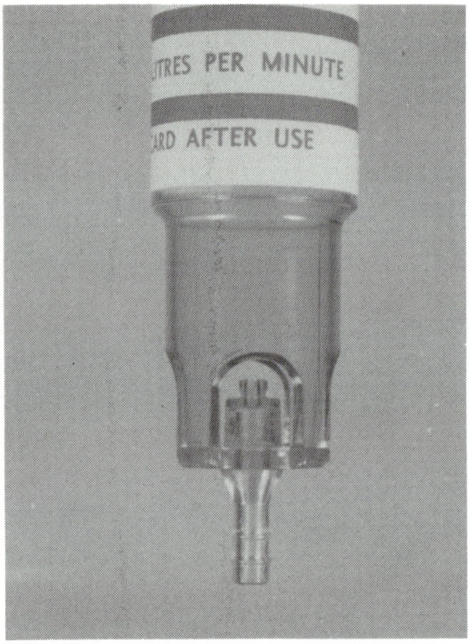

Fig. 5.7. *Close-up of "Ventimask" which uses the Venturi principle to give low concentrations of added inspired oxygen.*

(150 mmHg up to 175 mmHg) makes a difference to the patient's oxygenation because of the shape of the oxygen dissociation curve (see Fig. 5.3). A small rise in the P_aO_2 above 45 mmHg causes a marked rise in saturation. Once oxygen therapy has begun, regular assessment is necessary. If, after 30–60 minutes, there has been no increase in confusion or deterioration in level of consciousness one may try a slightly higher concentration of oxygen (i.e. 28%). If the patient does become more drowsy or confused, there is a strong suspicion that the P_aCO_2 has risen. Blood gas analysis should therefore be repeated. If the rise is not dramatic and the deterioration in consciousness does not progress rapidly, it may be justifiable to maintain that level of added oxygen, accepting a slightly higher P_aCO_2 as a necessary evil. Provided that other measures such as frequent physiotherapy and administration of antibiotics are instituted, the usual course is for the patient to gradually improve over the ensuing 12–24 hours. In some patients, the administration of added oxygen causes a rapidly progressive rise in P_aCO_2 with loss of consciousness. In these patients, the initial P_aCO_2 before commencement of oxygen treatment is usually 75

or 80 mmHg. When this situation arises the need for mechanical ventilation must be considered.

Measurement of blood gas tensions

Measurement of P_aCO_2 by the rebreathing technique

A most useful method of estimating arterial PCO_2 was described by Campbell and Howell (1962). In this method, the patient is connected via a mouthpiece and a tap system to a 2-litre bag containing 1·5 litres of pure oxygen (Fig. 5.8). The tap system enables the patient to breath from either the atmosphere or the bag, through the mouthpiece. A noseclip is used to obstruct the nostrils. The patient is seated comfortably and switched into rebreathing from the bag at the end of a normal expiration. The patient breathes normally and oxygen is taken up from the bag and nitrogen and carbon dioxide are eliminated into it. Rebreathing is continued for 1·5 minutes and then the tap is turned so that the contents of the bag are saved and the patient

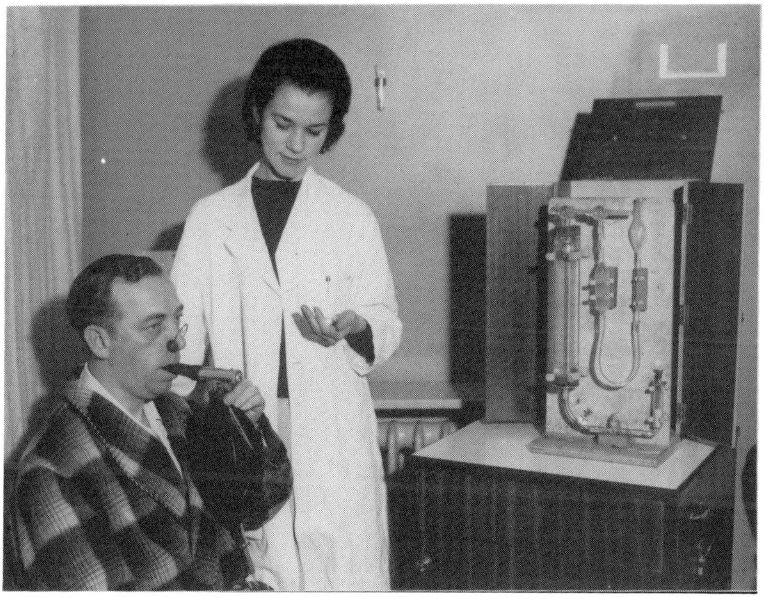

Fig. 5.8. *Measurement of* P_aCO_2 *by rebreathing technique.*

breathes from the atmosphere once more. The PCO_2 in the bag should have built up to a level approximately equal to the mixed venous PCO_2. If the PCO_2 in the bag is slightly higher than the mixed venous PCO_2 it may have caused a rise in P_aCO_2 and hence, eventually, a rise in mixed venous PCO_2. The period of breathing from the atmosphere is continued for two minutes so that the P_aCO_2 may return to normal, if it has risen. The patient is then again connected to the bag and rebreathes for a further 20 seconds. During this period, the PCO_2 in the bag either rises or falls slightly so as to equal the mixed venous PCO_2. There is not sufficient time in this 20 seconds for significant carbon dioxide retention to occur.

The concentration of carbon dioxide in the bag can now be measured. This is usually done using a Haldane apparatus which relies on the absorption of carbon dioxide by potassium hydroxide. While this is relatively simple to use, it yields reliable results. An infra-red absorption analyser is a useful alternative to the Haldane apparatus in laboratories with a high workload although this type of analyser is expensive. The PCO_2 in the bag, and hence the mixed venous PCO_2, can be calculated from the formula: $PCO_2 = \%CO_2/100 \times$ (barometric pressure minus 47 mmHg). In practice, $\%CO_2 \times 7$ is a useful approximation of this. The mixed venous PCO_2 is usually 6 mm higher than the arterial PCO_2. It is therefore customary to subtract 6 mm before expressing the result as "arterial PCO_2 obtained by rebreathing". In situations where there is a very high P_ACO_2, the difference between mixed venous and arterial PCO_2 may be rather more than 6 mmHg but the technique still gives a useful approximation. The advantage of this method is that it can be performed by relatively unskilled personnel and there is no need for arterial blood samples to be taken. Frequent measurements may therefore be taken at regular intervals in one patient without the need for multiple needle punctures.

Practical points

The initial volume of oxygen in the bag should not be too large—about three times tidal volume is correct. The patient must maintain an adequate tidal volume throughout the test. Leaks into the system will lower the result obtained and a certain amount of patient co-operation is required to avoid this. The technique can be used for unconscious patients by substituting a close-fitting face mask for the mouthpiece. We have used this technique in our laboratories for more than 15 years and have found it very useful in many situations where arterial puncture is not desirable. In particular it has been most reliable for the routine screening of patients before operations involving lung resection.

Blood gas analysis

The most widely used method of ascertaining the P_aCO_2 is by direct measurement on an arterial blood sample. This has the added advantage that other parameters such as arterial pH and P_aO_2 can also be measured.

Taking the sample

The technique of sampling blood from arteries is without risk provided care is taken and it is seldom more uncomfortable than a venepuncture. The best site is probably the radial artery provided that it has been established that the ulnar artery is adequate to supply the hand. This can be easily assessed by occluding both vessels at the wrist and then asking the patient to make a fist. On relaxing the fist, the hand will be pale and it will flush rapidly when the pressure on the ulnar artery alone is removed if this artery is adequate to supply the hand. Alternative sites are the brachial artery and femoral artery. Although thrombosis of these vessels would be catastrophic, it is fortunately very rare. A 2-ml syringe, preferably made of glass, is used. Initially 0·5 ml of heparin (1,000 units/ml) is drawn up and coated over the walls by moving the plunger up and down. All the air is then expelled, a fine needle attached, and the heparin expelled through it so that only the dead space of the syringe and the needle are filled with heparin. The chosen artery is palpated above and below the point of entry and the needle is then introduced in a nearly vertical manner. If a plastic syringe is being used, gentle suction can be applied all the time. With a glass syringe, the blood will enter the syringe when the arterial lumen is entered. Sometimes it is necessary to transfix the artery and then withdraw the needle exerting gentle suction on the plunger until blood appears in the syringe. Occasionally, if repeated samples will be required, it is wise to insert an in-dwelling catheter into the artery, the radial and femoral arteries being the most popular sites. This is generally a matter for someone with considerable experience of the technique and will not be described here.

In some instances arterial puncture may not be feasible. So-called "arterialised" blood can be obtained from the vasodilated ear lobe by pricking and collection in a capillary tube. An oximeter can also be applied to the vasodilated ear to give information on oxygen saturation *only*. These methods are less satisfactory than arterial blood gas analyses and require specialised equipment.

Machines for performing blood gas analysis

Detailed consideration of the types of machine available for use in blood gas analysis and of their operation is beyond the scope of this book. However, the following short discussion may prove a useful introduction to the topic.

There are two main methods for measuring carbon dioxide tensions in blood. One of these involves a direct-reading carbon dioxide electrode. This requires skillful care for the production of accurate results but in general is easy to use. The other technique uses the Astrup microelectrode for pH measurement in association with tonometry of the blood with two different gas mixtures of known carbon dioxide tension. The results can be read off the Siggaard-Andersen nomogram. This method is fairly straightforward but is slightly more time consuming and subject to several sources of error including inaccurate measurement of pH and inefficient equilibration with the standardised gases.

Blood pH level is measured with a glass direct-reading pH electrode. Oxygen tension and oxygen content of the blood can be measured using oxygen electrodes and the Van Slyke apparatus.

All of these types of apparatus need careful maintenance and attention, preferably from one member of staff only, be it doctor or technician. This person should have attended a course run by the manufacturer of the machine and be fully conversant with simple maintenance and repairs. The machines should also be calibrated at least twice a day if accurate results are to be obtained. A number of automated machines are now available, but they still need careful technical supervision.

Interpretation of blood gas analysis results

Although blood gas analysis is widely performed, the interpretation of the results is often inadequate. The information obtained by the specialist from the analysis of blood gases can, however, be very great.

Here we will not concern ourselves with complex physiological calculations but simply consider blood gases in the clinical context.

Arterial pH. The measurement of arterial pH can give valuable information. The normal value is 7·42 plus/minus 0·02 and deviations from this may have either metabolic or respiratory causes. Compensatory effects may also occur. Thus the patient with status asthmaticus who goes into acute respiratory failure with rising P_aCO_2 may have a low pH of say, 7·24. The patient with chronic bronchitis may have the same level of P_aCO_2 but because of the chronic nature of the condition, sufficient time will have passed for renal retention of bicarbonate to develop and the arterial pH may be normal. Similarly, a patient with pyloric stenosis who has been vomiting for several days may be alkalotic, but CO_2 retention will occur and the arterial pH may be deceptively normal (Davenport, 1969).

Arterial PCO_2. The P_aCO_2 measurement is the most widely used and useful of all our measurements. The P_aCO_2 is kept in the range of 35–45 mmHg quite constantly in the normal subject, any rise above this leading to marked dyspnoea and discomfort. The two factors affecting the P_aCO_2 are the rate of production of carbon dioxide, and its rate of elimination by the lungs. This elimination can be related to the amount of *alveolar* ventilation (see above). These relationships are shown diagrammatically in Fig. 5.9. Clearly, if production of carbon dioxide rises with no change in alveolar ventilation, the P_aCO_2 will rise. Similarly, hypoventilation with constant carbon dioxide production will also cause a rise in P_aCO_2. This simple relationship is the key to understanding changes in P_aCO_2. Apart from those conditions in which there is a very high metabolic rate, the P_aCO_2 is normally inversely proportional to the amount of alveolar ventilation. This must not be confused with *minute* ventilation (see Chapter 2). Alveolar ventilation may be reduced because of diminished respiratory drive, as occurs in chronic bronchitis or the exhaustion stage of status asthmaticus, or by the effect of drugs. Measurement of the P_aCO_2 is the only practical way that information about alveolar ventilation can be obtained. Clinical observation or measurement of minute ventilation of the mouth are quite useless in this respect. Quite simply, a rising P_aCO_2 means that alveolar ventilation is, for whatever reason, becom-

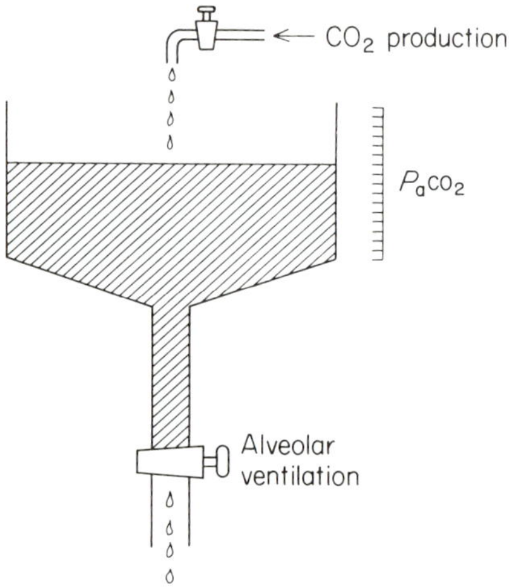

Fig. 5.9. *Analogy of CO_2 production and alveolar ventilation with water tank.* P_aCO_2 *will rise if CO_2 production increases or if alveolar ventilation decreases.*

ing inadequate and that respiratory failure is commencing. The application of this information is discussed in the clinical examples below.

Arterial P_aO_2. The normal P_aO_2 is 80–100 mmHg. P_aO_2 may be reduced by several mechanisms. For example, there may be insufficient ventilation of perfused alveoli, in which case the $\dot{V}_A/\dot{Q}$ abnormality will lead to a "shunt" effect, or there may be an actual anatomical right-to-left shunt as occurs in some congenital heart disease. Further, if the P_aCO_2 is high, the P_aO_2 must be low if the patient is breathing air. Normally the sum of the gas tensions for oxygen and carbon dioxide in the arterial blood equals 130–150 mmHg. If the sum of these two gas tensions is less than this, a significant degree of shunting from right to left is occurring.

Cyanosis is usually apparent when P_aO_2 is less than 50 mmHg but it may appear at a higher P_aO_2 if the patient is polycythaemic or it may not be present even at quite low levels of P_aO_2 if the patient is very anaemic.

Clinical examples of the application of information obtained from blood gas analysis

Asthma. The asthmatic patient usually has quite normal blood gas levels between attacks. When an episode of asthma begins, the asthmatic generally hyperventilates and the P_aCO_2 falls, often to around 30 mmHg. The P_aO_2 may be normal or just below normal at this stage. In a mild attack, this situation will continue until the patient returns to normal. If the attacks persists, however, the patient may develop more severe bronchospasm and become rather tired. Respiratory effort will be reduced and, as the airways resistance rises, it will become less effective in maintaining alveolar ventilation. This means that the P_aCO_2 will rise, but initially only into the normal range again. The P_aO_2 may fall further but the patient will probably still not appear cyanosed.

Mrs M. S., aged 32, suffered a cold for four days prior to admission to hospital. Breathlessness began two days before admission. She was awake all night with severe breathlessness the night before and was very anxious and restless on admission when the following results were obtained: pH, 7·40; P_aCO_2, 42 mmHg; P_aO_2, 75 mmHg. These results are virtually normal. The history would suggest, however, that she has been suffering from acute severe asthma for some 24–36 hours and her P_aCO_2 was probably well below 35 mmHg 12 hours before admission. The slight decrease in P_aO_2 was not at first sight worrying but the situation needed careful watching. Far from complacently accepting these results as nearly normal, the doctors looking after this woman began enthusiastic treatment with steroids, antibiotics, bronchodilators and physiotherapy and repeated the blood gas tests 3 hours later when pH = 7·35, P_aCO_2 = 50 mmHg and P_aO_2 = 60 mmHg. At this stage, the patient was still not cyanosed and her respiratory effort still appeared adequate. The rising P_aCO_2, however, showed that she had reduced her alveolar ventilation and was now in respiratory failure. This is a very sinister stage for an asthmatic and soon after these results were obtained she was transferred to an intensive therapy unit and mechanical ventilation was started. Some of the possibilities of change in arterial levels of carbon dioxide tension in asthma are shown diagrammatically in Fig. 5.10.

Thus a normal P_aCO_2 in an asthmatic who has been in an acute, severe attack and does not seem to be improving, demands further assessment very promptly to ascertain whether the P_aCO_2 is still rising. Intensive treatment short of mechanical ventilation may well avert the onset of respiratory failure but, if the patient becomes too exhausted, mechanical ventilation must be considered.

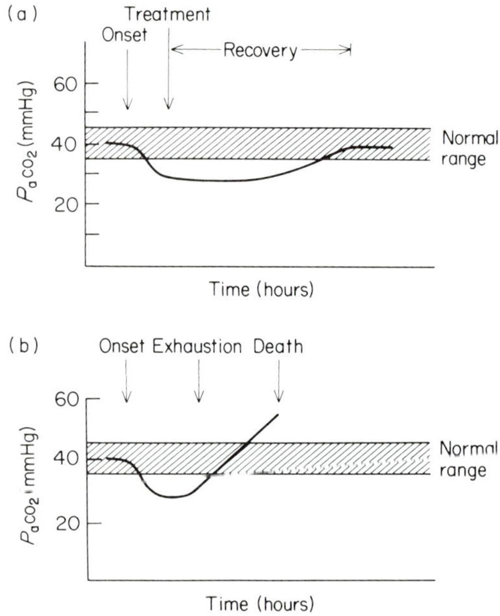

Fig. 5.10. *Blood gas changes in asthma. An apparently normal* P_aCO_2 *level in the presence of an acute attack may indicate impending exhaustion: (a) successfully treated case, (b) possible result of failure to treat.*

Chronic Bronchitis. It is well known that the patient with chronic bronchitis tends to go into respiratory and cardiac failure at a relatively early stage of the disease. It is because of this that such patients are sometimes known as "blue bloaters".

Mr G. K., aged 58, had suffered a chronic cough with sputum production for eight years. He had been a very heavy smoker in past years and still smoked 10 cigarettes per day. When assessed initially in the lung function laboratory his blood gas measurements were as follows: pH, 7·41; P_aCO_2, 60 mmHg; P_aO_2, 55 mmHg. At this time, he was feeling reasonably well, was not too breathless to get around and was managing a desk job. Some months later, during the winter, he was admitted to hospital having developed severe breathlessness associated with the production of purulent sputum. On admission his blood gas measurements were as follows: pH, 7·38; P_aCO_2, 72 mmHg; P_aO_2, 35 mmHg. He appeared obviously cyanosed and in view of the low P_aO_2 he was given 24% oxygen. During the night after his admission, regular arousal and physiotherapy were performed and he was given antibiotics and bronchodilators. After two hours of oxygen therapy, his P_aCO_2 had risen to 78 mmHg and his P_aO_2 had risen to 48 mmHg. He was slightly confused but his clinical situation did not deteriorate during the night and within 48 hours of admission his blood gases had nearly returned to the same levels as when he was first seen in the outpatients department. Attempting to manage a patient like this in respiratory failure and to administer oxygen is extremely difficult without help from blood gas analysis. Serial measurements of the mixed venous PCO_2 by the rebreathing technique can be useful in this situation, especially if the skilled personnel who operate blood gas analysis machines are not available.

Emphysema. Mr K. H., aged 57, had suffered progressive breathlessness over the last 8 years with occasional chest infections but no constantly productive cough or other symptom. At the time of presentation he had had symptoms for five years and his blood gas measurements were as follows: pH, 7·44; P_aCO_2, 30 mmHg; P_aO_2, 85 mmHg. At this time, his P_aCO_2 was low indicating alveolar hyperventilation and P_aO_2 was normal. This man would fit into the class of patient known as "pink puffers". Now, three years later, this man's breathlessness is much worse and he has suffered several episodes of right-sided heart failure. His blood gases are now as follows: pH, 7·40; P_aCO_2, 50 mmHg; P_aO_2, 60 mmHg. The situation has changed in that he is now in early respiratory failure and has some reduction in his arterial oxygen tension. Carbon dioxide retention and heart failure are relatively late features in emphysema when compared with chronic bronchitis. This man died from emphysema four months after these blood gas tensions were measured.

Drug Overdosage. Miss K. D., aged 18, was admitted as an emergency, having been found unconscious at home. It was believed that she had taken barbiturate sleeping tablets in overdose but the time at which she took them was unknown. On admission, she was deeply unconscious and barely maintaining a clear airway. Blood gas analyses were performed, and the results were: pH, 7·38; PCO_2, 54 mmHg; PO_2, 50 mmHg. These results clearly indicated that she was in respiratory failure and that the drug had had a sufficiently depressant effect on her respiratory centre to reduce alveolar ventilation markedly. She was intubated and mechanical ventilation commenced without delay.

It can not be over-emphasized that measurement of minute volume at the mouth with a Wright's anemometer can be very misleading in these cases and that usually several estimations of arterial blood gases are required to ensure that the situation is not deteriorating.

References

Campbell, E. J. M. and Howell, J. B. L. (1962). A rebreathing method for estimating the mixed venous carbon dioxide tension. *British Medical Journal* **2**, 630–631.

Donald, K. W., Renzetti, A., Riley, R. L. and Cournand, A. (1952). Analysis of factors affecting concentration of oxygen and carbon dioxide in gas and blood of lungs. *J. Appl. Physiol.* **4**, 497–525.

Davenport, H. W. (1969). *The ABC of Acid Base Chemistry*. 5th Ed. Chicago: Univ. Chicago Press.

-6- Diffusion

The function of the lungs is gas exchange. This ultimately occurs in the alveoli where oxygen and carbon dioxide (and other gases) pass across the so-called alveolar–capillary membrane separating the alveolar air space from the pulmonary capillary blood. This may present a physically minute barrier (see Fig. 5.2). The passage of the physiologically important gases, oxygen and carbon dioxide is by simple diffusion which is in turn related to the partial pressures of the gases on either side of the membrane. The difficulty in attempting to measure this diffusion of gas (and in particular that of oxygen) is that of obtaining samples truly representing *alveolar* gas and *pulmonary capillary* blood. Obviously sampling individual alveolar units would be impractical. Sampling expired air (however collected) provides information only on the gas content of a mixture of air expired from multiple alveoli plus dead space. Furthermore, in disease, there may be gross mis-matching of air and blood flow (ventilation/perfusion inequality—see Chapter 2) so that a group of alveoli may have little or no blood flow, yet plenty of air flow and vice versa. Indeed the whole process of gas transfer can be compared to a man in London using the underground railway (Table 6.1).

Despite the difficulties involved, attempts have been made to determine the efficiency of the lungs in taking up oxygen and indeed to measure their so-called diffusing capacity. Such measurements have of necessity been rather indirect. Most have employed carbon monoxide (CO) as the test gas rather than oxygen. There have been several reasons for this. Historically Marie Krogh (1915) chose this gas because at that time there was no doubt that it entered the pul-

Table 6.1. *Analogy between use of London underground railway and oxygen transfer*

	Railway use		Gas transfer	
Step	Process	Possible difficulties	Process	Possible difficulties
1	Man descends escalator toward platform	Escalator may be blocked by luggage etc.	O_2 passes down airway toward alveolus	Airway may be blocked by tenacious sputum or bronchoconstriction
2	Man stands on platform	Platform may be too small for crowd or not be supplied with rail-way line	O_2 enters alveolus	Alveolus may be collapsed or fibrosed (i.e. not ventilated—no room for gas) or may not be associated with blood capillary

3	Train arrives	Train may not arrive	Blood circulates in capilliary	Blood supply may fail e.g. following pulmonary embolus or in cough syncope (alveolus not perfused)
4	Man enters train through doors	Doors may fail to open fully slowing passage into train (especially bad effect during rush hour)	O_2 passes across alveolar–capilliary membrane into the blood	Fibrosis of membrane may slow rate of O_2 transfer (especially noticeable on exercise with increased ventilation)
5	Man finds seat	Most or all seats may be occupied and man ∴ unable to travel (no standing allowed)	O_2 combines with haemoglobin (Hb)	Hb mechanism may be upset e.g. in CO poisoning
6	Full train pulls away	Train may not move away properly	Oxygenated blood moves on	Blood flow may be sluggish as in heart failure

monary capillaries by diffusion (there were still some workers proposing the *secretion* of oxgyen from the alveoli into the blood at that time), and also because there was no doubt that *before* its inhalation into the lungs the concentration of carbon monoxide in the blood would be zero. Other advantages are:

1. Carbon monoxide combines with haemoglobin more readily and rapidly than oxygen, and its use *reduces* any effect of the chemical combination of the test gas with haemoglobin;
2. There is no metabolism or use of carbon monoxide in the lung itself;
3. It is very easy to analyse carbon monoxide concentration accurately and rapidly.

Because the molecular weight of carbon monoxide (28) is fairly similar to that of oxygen (32) its diffusing properties across the alveolar–capilliary membrane are similar to those of oxygen. In fact it is now customary to measure the diffusing capacity of carbon monoxide (D_LCO) only. This can easily be converted to a diffusing capacity for oxygen, although it is not usual to do so.

Measurement of diffusing capacity

While a detailed discussion of all the methods of measuring diffusing capacity is beyond the scope of this book, they will be described briefly below. These methods fall into two main classes, those involving a breath holding manoeuvre and those involving "steady-state" measurements. Each class has its advantages and disadvantages as the Kroghs found out as long ago as 1910. In Great Britain and Europe most workers use a breath holding technique whilst in America, the steady-state methods are more popular.

Single breath method

This is really a refinement of Marie Krogh's breath holding method. The use of helium obviates the necessity of obtaining *two* samples of expired air to determine the mean alveolar carbon monoxide concentration. The test is carried out by asking subjects to inhale air containing a mixture of carbon monoxide (CO: about 0·028%) and

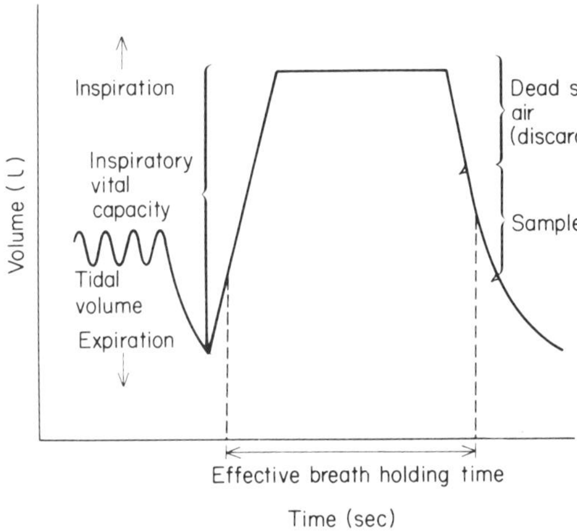

Fig. 6.1. *Spirographic trace illustrating transfer factor measurement. The subject breathes out as much as possible (to residual volume) and then inhales fully and holds the breath for about 10 seconds. He then expires and, after discarding the first 600 ml as "dead space air" a sample of the expired gas is taken for analysis.*

helium (He: 10%) by taking in as deep a breath as possible (maximum *inspiratory* vital capacity (IVC) see Fig. 6.1). The breath is then held for 10 seconds and expired forcibly. The initial 600 ml of expirate is discarded as "dead space air" and a sample of the rest is analysed for carbon monoxide and helium content. The dilution of helium is used in two ways. Firstly, it is used as a "10 second single breath" helium washout to estimate total lung capacity (TLC), or more precisely breath holding volume, from the IVC measured from the trace. Secondly, it is used as an estimate of the degree of dilution of the inspired carbon monoxide when distributed thoughout the whole lung.

Thus: (1) Breath holding volume (V_A) $= \text{IVC} \times \text{He}_I/\text{He}_E$

and (2) Corrected "whole lung" inspired CO concentration (F_ICO) $= \text{CO}_I \times \text{He}_E/\text{He}_I$

where He_I = helium concentration in inspired gas
He_E = helium concentration in expired gas
CO_I = carbon monoxide concentration in inspired gas

The apparatus can be made from an appropriate spirometer, a

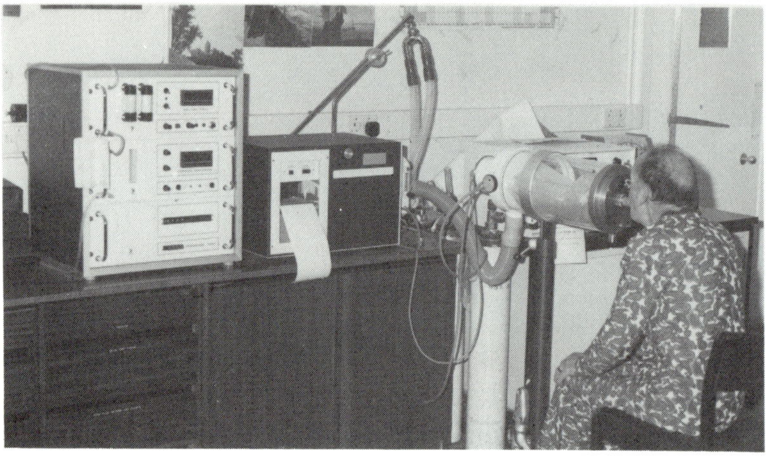

Fig. 6.2. *Single breath transfer factor apparatus in use.*

bag-in-bottle, and a 3-way valve. The manoeuvre can be standardised by using electronic control of the gas collection and timing and appropriate apparatus—the Resparameter "Transfer Test" (Fig. 6.2) is now available commercially in the U.K. through P. K. Morgan. The tests make a number of assumptions, not least that inspired gas is distributed rapidly and evenly throughout the lungs, particularly to the gas exchanging alveoli. They also assume that there is a reasonable matching of blood and gas flow. Such a perfect distribution and ventilation/perfusion balance is barely achieved in the healthy lung, much less in the presence of disease.

For these reasons, in the U.K. and throughout Europe the name of the test has been changed from the diffusion test to the gas transfer test and the measurement from diffusing capacity (D_LCO) to transfer factor (T_L). The old units were ml/mmHg/min which can be converted to the new S.I. units of mmol min^{-1} kPa^{-1} by multiplication by a factor of 0.335 (see Appendix 1).

$$T_L = xV_A\left(t \times \log_{10}\left[\frac{F_I\text{CO}}{F_E\text{CO}}\right]\right)$$

Where x = 160*

t = The effective breath holding time

*For derivation of x, which includes factors for converting from STPD to BTPS and from $\log_e$ to $\log_{10}$ see Cotes 1979 (pp. 242–243).

V_A = Alveolar volume or breath holding volume
F_ICO = Initial "whole lung" CO concentration
F_ECO = CO concentration in expired sample

In carrying out the test, attention to detail is important. This applies to many aspects, including the calibration of the gas analysers and the standardisation of the volume and breath holding times. Full discussion of these is not within the scope of this book but the reader is referred to Forster (1964), Ogilvie *et al.* (1957), Jones and Meade (1961) and Cotes (1963). There are also excellent reviews in books by Cotes (1979) and Bates, Macklem and Christie (1971).

Further refinements of the test are possible. The total transfer factor includes the alveolar volume (V_A) in the numerator, and so is dependent on lung size. One may be more interested in carbon monoxide transfer per unit of unit volume or transfer coefficient (K_{CO}) as it is called. The two are related as follows:–

$$T_L = V_A \times K_{CO}$$

or

$$K_{CO} = T_L/V_A$$

Many believe that K_{CO} is a more meaningful measurement than T_L (e.g. McGrath and Thompson, 1969). In that one may want to estimate the total gas transfer as well as that per unit of lung volume, it may be more appropriate to estimate both T_L and K_{CO}.

By making measurements of carbon monoxide transfer at different levels of oxygen concentration, it is possible to sub-divide the transfer factor into two components, the diffusing capacity of the membrane (D_M) and the capillary blood volume (V_C). These are related as follows: $1/T_L = 1/D_M \neq 1/\theta V_C$ where θ is the volume of gas (in ml) which will be taken up by the red cells in 1 ml of blood per min per mmHg gradient of pressure between the plasma and the red cell. This concept is quite complicated and was largely developed by Roughton and Forster (1957) and applied as a clinical physiological test by Lewis *et al.* (1958). In fact, considerable precision in making the measurements, especially that of T_L breathing 100% oxygen is required and results have not always been found easy to reproduce. Patients have not always been ready to accept multiple measurements and the test has, in fact, not been applied widely.

Although there remains criticism of the measurement of the

single breath diffusing capacity (transfer factor), it has been found a useful test clinically to detect impairment of function in diseases causing widespread fibrosis of the lung (e.g. fibrosing alveolitis, asbestosis) and has been increasingly used as an objective measurement in assessing disability resulting from industrial lung disease. Furthermore, serial studies may reveal either the progression and natural history of the disease (e.g. asbestosis) or its improvement with treatment (e.g. sarcoidosis). It has become an accepted measurement and is performed increasingly in Europe and North America.

Steady state methods

These methods involve measuring the rate of carbon monoxide uptake during continuous breathing. The main difficulty here lies in the estimation of the dead space (V_D) which has a very different value in rapid shallow breathing to that in normal breathing. Initially, Krogh (1915) tried using assumed dead space values to derive the *alveolar* carbon monoxide concentration. She found that this concentration varied considerably with changes in tidal volume (V_T) due to undue sensitivity to changes in physiological dead space that occurred when the ratio of V_D to V_T changed. Attempts to define V_D more accurately have involved simultaneous measurement of arterial $P\text{CO}_2$ suggested by Filley *et al.* (1954) and *end-tidal* $P\text{CO}_2$ (Marshall, 1958). End-tidal sampling is not always easy and satisfactory, however, especially during exercise, when the sample becomes less representative of the mean alveolar gas.

These methods do not require helium analysis and are *relatively* simple. They are to some extent dependent on the ventilation and may give falsely low values of T_L due to the use of a non-representative alveolar sample. The interpretation of the results may be difficult. A normal result certainly excludes serious lung diseases but spuriously low values may be produced as explained above.

Other methods

Other methods include a rebreathing method which neccessitates continuous monitoring of the carbon monoxide and helium concentrations in a rebreathing circuit. A correlation must be made for the concentration of carbon monoxide saturated haemoglobin. In addition, some hyperventilation occurs due to accumulation carbon dioxide.

Detailed discussion of these methods is beyond the scope of this book but they are described, criticised and compared in a simple table in Chapter 2 of Bates, Macklem and Christie (1971).

Interpretation of results

Much could be written on the interpretation of transfer factor measurements. The first point to be made is the problem of normal values. The most appropriate ones are provided by Cotes (1979), but it should be remembered that real racial differences may exist and that there is still some controversy about whether there is any difference in the changes produced by ageing in men and women respectively (Cotes and Hall, 1970). It is also necessary to make a correction for the concentration of haemoglobin in the blood. The results obtained in any patient should be adjusted to a standard haemoglobin concentration of 14·6 g/l and an alveolar oxygen tension of 120 mmHg* (Cotes and Hall, 1968). This is rarely done in clinical practice, however. The correction for haemoglobin concentration is important if significant anaemia is present.

The relatively large list of references at the end of this chapter reflects the intricacies involved in measurements of gas transfer. The test is nevertheless clinically useful in that T_L will be reduced in a number of illnesses leading to diffuse pulmonary fibrosis (see Chapter 9). Finding such a reduction in transfer factor can be an important element in the diagnosis. It is also reduced in emphysema (see Chapter 7) and this reduction can help to distinguish emphysema from asthma and bronchitis.

References

Bates, D. V., Maklem, P. T. and Christie, R. V. (1971). *Respiratory Function in Disease*. 2nd Ed. London: W. B. Saunders.

*For conversion to SI units see Appendix 1.

Cotes, J. E. (1963). Effect of variability in gas analysis on the reproducibility of the pulmonary diffusing capacity by the single breath method. *Thorax* **18**, 151–154.

Cotes, J. E. (1979). *Lung Function: Assessment and Application in Medicine.* 4th Ed. London: Blackwell Scientific Publications.

Cotes, J. E. and Hall, A. M. (1968). The effect of a change in haemoglobin concentration upon the lung transfer factor for carbon monoxide of normal subjects. *Bull. Physio-Pathol. Resp.* **4**, 691–693.

Cotes, J. E. and Hall, A. M. (1970). The transfer factor of the lung: Normal values in adults. *Normal Values for Respiratory Function in Man—A Symposium.* Panminerva Medica. Pp. 327–344.

Filley, G. F., Macintosh, D. J. and Wright, G. W. (1954). Carbon monoxide uptake and pulmonary diffusing capacity in normal subjects at rest and during exercise. *J. clin. Invest.* **33**, 530–539.

Forster, R. E. (1964). Interpretation of measurements of pulmonary diffusing capacity. *Handbook of Physiology, Section 3, Respiration* **2**, 1453–1455.

Jones, R. S. and Meade, F. (1961). A theoretical and experimental analysis of abnormalities in estimations of pulmonary diffusing capacity by the single breath method. *Q. J. Exp. Physiol.* **46**, 131–143.

Krogh, M. (1915). The diffusion of gases through the lungs of man. *J. Physiol.* **49**, 271–300.

Lewis, B. M., Lin, T. H., Noe, F. E. and Komisaruk, R. (1958). The measurement of pulmonary capillary blood volume and pulmonary membrane diffusing capacity in normal subjects; the effects of exercise and position. *J. clin. Invest.* **37**, 1061–1070.

McGrath, M. W. and Thomson, M. L. (1959). The effect of age, body size and lung volume change on alveolar–capillary permeability and diffusing capacity in man. *J. Physiol.* **146**, 572–582.

Marshall, R. (1958). A comparison of methods for measuring the diffusing capacity of the lungs for carbon monoxide. Investigation by fractional analysis of alveolar air. *J. clin. Invest.* **37**, 394–408.

Ogilivie, C. M., Forster, R. E., Blakemore, W. S. and Morton, J. W. (1957). A standardized breath-holding technique for the clinical measurement of the diffusing capacity of the lung for carbon monoxide. *J. clin. Invest.* **36**, 1–7.

Roughton, F. J. W. and Forster, R. E. (1957). Relative importance of diffusion and chemical reaction rates in determining the rate of exchange of gases in the human lung, with special reference to true diffusing capacity of pulmonary membrane and volume of blood in lung capillaries. *J. appl. Physiol.* **11**, 290–302.

-7- Further parameters and tests of lung function

So far, we have considered rather simple tests which are frequently performed in lung function laboratories, and have seen how much useful information can be derived from them in clinical situations. The fact that these tests are simple to perform, however, does not mean that their underlying mechanisms are straightforward; they are indirect ways of drawing conclusions about changes in very basic properties of the lungs which are themselves rather tedious to actually measure. These properties are the *lung elastic recoil pressure* and the *resistance* of the airways. We shall consider these in more detail and also give an account of some of the less standard tests which the well-equipped lung function laboratory can now perform.

Lung elastic recoil pressure

If a balloon is attached to a syringe and partially inflated, a pressure has to be exerted on the syringe plunger to keep the balloon at a constant volume (Fig. 7.1a). If the syringe plunger is being held still, clearly the pressure being exerted on it is exactly balanced by an opposite pressure resulting from the distended balloon tending to deflate and return to its resting collapsed state. This pressure is the elastic recoil pressure of the balloon at that volume. If the syringe plunger is further depressed, the balloon will inflate to a larger volume, and a greater pressure must be exerted on the plunger to keep the balloon inflated (Fig. 7.1b). Clearly, the balloon's elastic recoil pressure is now greater at this larger volume and this balances exactly

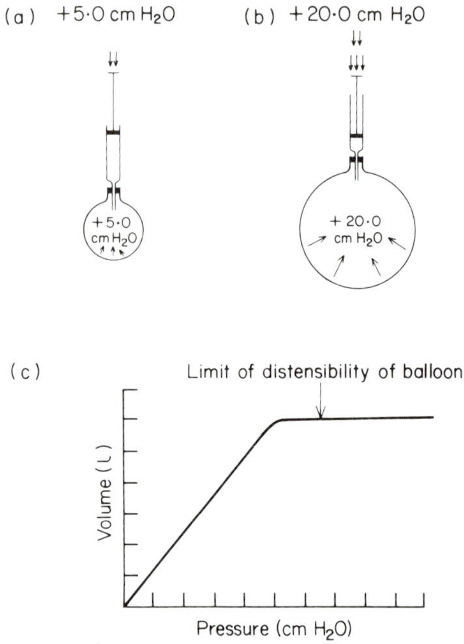

Fig. 7.1. *Relationship between volume and pressure in inflation of a balloon (see text for explanation).*

the increased pressure being exerted on the syringe plunger. The relationship of pressure needed to distend the balloon, and the resulting volume can be expressed graphically (Fig. 7.1c), the resulting line having a slope equal to the ratio of the change in volume to the corresponding change in pressure. This slope is called the *compliance* of the balloon. A balloon which is very stiff and hard to inflate will have a low compliance and the slope of the line in the graph will be rather flat; a balloon which is very soft and easy to inflate will have a high compliance and the line will be rather steep. The units of compliance will be l/cmH_2O. Figure 7.1c shows that the pressure–volume relationship becomes non-linear at higher volumes; here the balloon is more difficult to distend and thus the compliance becomes very low.

The lungs resemble this simple system with the important difference that the distending pressure is not usually a positive pressure applied at the mouth, but a negative pressure in the pleural cavities

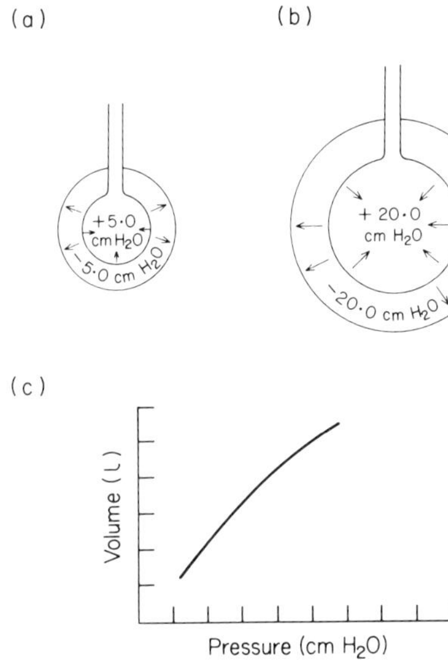

Fig. 7.2. *Relationship between volume and pressure in inflation of the lung (see text for explanation).*

surrounding the lung. The only frequently occurring situation in which a positive pressure is applied at the mouth is during artificial ventilation.

At the end of a quiet expiration, the lungs are at the *functional residual capacity*. This volume is determined by the exact balance of the forces affecting the pressure in the pleural cavity (the tendency of the ribs to spring outwards) and the lung elastic recoil pressure (the tendency of the lungs to collapse inwards as shown in Figure 7.2a, as a result of the contraction of stretched elastic fibres in the lung parenchyma and of surface tension forces in the alveoli).

If the muscles of inspiration pull the ribs outwards and upwards and make the pleural cavity pressure more negative, the lungs will inflate just as the balloon did in the example above. If the breath is then held, a new equilibrium is set up with a higher lung elastic recoil pressure at the larger lung volume (Fig. 7.2b). Thus a pressure–volume curve can be constructed for the lung, and the slope of this curve will be a measure of static lung compliance (Fig. 7.2c).

Measurement of compliance

To measure compliance in practice, it is necessary to record simultaneously changes in volume and transpulmonary pressure. Volume changes can easily be recorded using a spirometer. Transpulmonary pressure is usually measured as the difference between pressure within the oesophagus and pressure within the mouth. To record oesophageal pressure, a fine tube, the end of which is protected by a balloon containing a small amount of air, is passed into the oesphagus so that its tip lies 45 cms from the mouth. The recording end of this tube is connected to a differential pressure transducer and the opposite side of this transducer is connected to the mouthpiece. With appropriate electrical circuitry it is possible to record directly on an X–Y recorder the changes which occur in volume and transpulmonary pressure (Fig. 7.3), (Milic-Emili *et al.*, 1964).

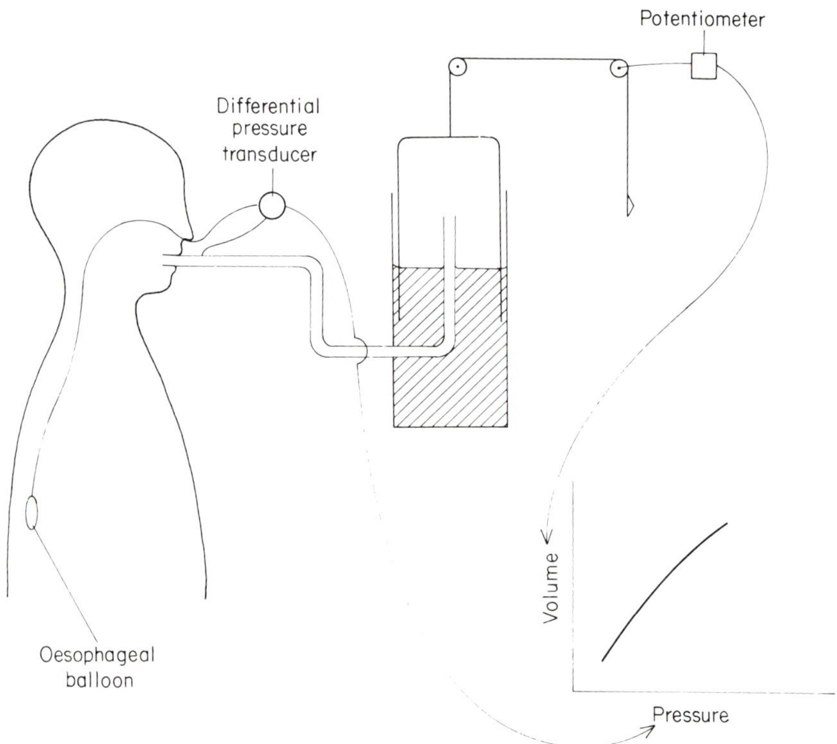

Fig. 7.3. *Measurement of compliance.*

After performing a standard volume history (e.g. three deep breaths) the subject takes a deep breath in and begins to exhale slowly. As the amount of air in the lungs decreases towards residual volume, a shutter is put across the mouthpiece every 300 ml or so and kept in place for a few seconds whilst transpulmonary pressure is recorded on the X–Y trace. This gives a pressure–volume trace from which compliance can be derived. In practice, the measurement of compliance is a difficult procedure in which the operator is required to pay great attention to detail. It is not useful as a test in the general laboratory. Increased compliance may be seen in patients with emphysema and decreased compliance may be present in patients with obesity and with pulmonary fibrosis. However, the wide variation in compliance among normal, healthy subjects makes interpretation of small changes rather difficult.

Airway resistance

The concept of resistance of tubes is a rather simple one. It is easy to see from Fig. 7.4 that to achieve the same flow rate through the narrower as through the wider tube, a greater pressure has to be applied at one end. If the same pressure is applied at the end of both tubes, the resultant flow rate will therefore be lower in the narrower tube. Although a similar principle applies to the bronchi, the situation is made much more complex by the continual branching nature of the airways, and the difficulties of interpreting the combination of laminar and turbulent flow. Nevertheless, airway resistance is one of the factors that affects changes in measurements of such factors as the forced expired volume in one second or the peak expiratory flow rate.

Direct measurement of airway resistance is really a procedure for the research physiologist because the most satisfactory equipment (the body plethysmograph) is delicate and expensive. Using this technique, the resistance of the airways can be fairly easily measured and three points are worthy of note here:

1. The recording of airway resistance is done while the subject is gently panting. This means that full inflation and forced expiration are not required. This is sometimes very useful when studying asthmatic patients in whom these manoeuvres may induce bron-

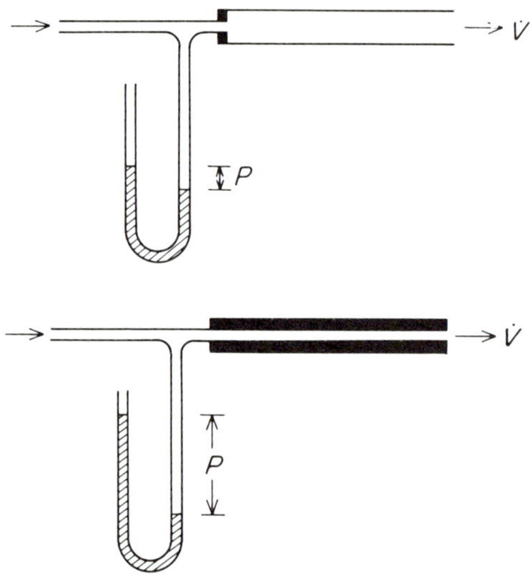

Fig. 7.4. *Differences in applied pressure required to pass the same flow of gas through (a) a wide tube and (b) a narrow tube.*

chospasm, or when looking for small effects of drugs where the measurements themselves should not change broncho-motor tone.

2. Airway resistance (R_{aw}) is related in a curvilinear manner to lung volume, but the reciprocal of resistance, airway conductance (G_{aw}), is related to lung volume in a linear manner (Fig. 7.5). This makes correction for volume differences between measurements much easier and many authors use specific conductance (SG_{aw}) to express their results. This is the slope of the conductance–volume plot and thus changes in specific conductance will indicate true changes in airway calibre rather than changes in lung volume (Dubois *et al.*, 1956).
3. The bulk of the resistance of the airways is in the larynx, trachea and larger bronchi. If the normal airway resistance is 2·0 cm H_2O/l/sec, then 1·8 cm H_2O/l/sec of this will be from large airways and 0·2 cm H_2O/l/sec will be from the smaller bronchi (less than 5 mm diameter). This means the changes in the calibre of the smaller airways have to be relatively large to produce any measurable rise in airway resistance, and that if large changes in airway resistance do occur they are probably resulting from narrowing of the larger airways.

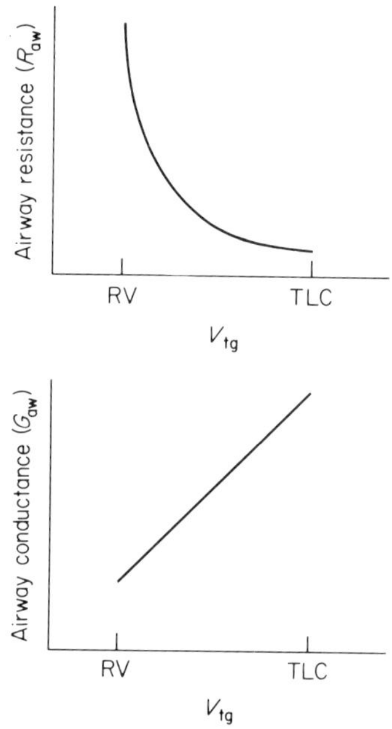

Fig. 7.5 *(a) Relationship of airway resistance* (R_{aw}) *to thoracic gas volume* (V_{tg}). *(b) Relationship of conductance* (G_{aw}) *to* V_{tg}. *Slope of line is the specific conductance* (SG_{aw}).

It is beyond the scope of this book to describe in detail the technique of measurement of airway resistance using the body plethysmograph, but the points mentioned above should be useful to the reader when interpreting papers in which airway resistance or its derivatives are reported.

Flow rate

Although the equipment necessary for recording flow rates is rather expensive, these measurements are widely used in many laboratories, and many publications report the results of their use. Certainly, they have their advantages, but their application in clinical practice and research is not straight-forward. Before considering flow rate in detail, it is helpful to introduce the concept of flow limitation.

Flow limitation

In Fig. 7.6, the alveoli are represented by a circle, the airways by a single tube and the chest wall by a box. Figure 7.6a shows the situation which occurs when there is no inspiratory or expiratory effort. The glottis is open and the pressure in the alveoli, the airways and the

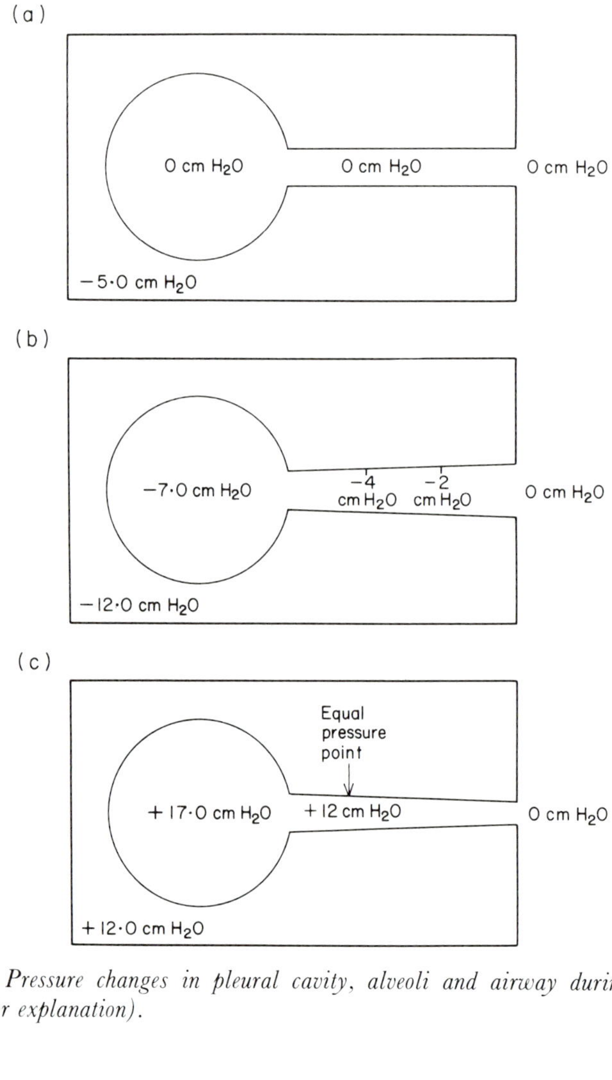

Fig. 7.6. *Pressure changes in pleural cavity, alveoli and airway during breathing (see text for explanation).*

mouth is atmospheric (zero). The alveoli are kept open by a distending, negative intrapleural pressure of $-5{\cdot}0$ cm H_2O which exactly balances the elastic recoil pressure of the lung. During inspiration (Fig. 7.6b), the intrapleural pressure falls further to $12{\cdot}0$ cm H_2O and a pressure gradient is set up between the alveoli and the mouth. In the alveoli, pressure is the sum of intrapleural pressure and elastic recoil pressure of the lung ($-12{\cdot}0$ cm H_2O and $+5{\cdot}0$ cm H_2O) that is $-7{\cdot}0$ cm H_2O. The airways within the chest tend to be rather expanded because of the distending negative pressure around them. During forced expiration, however (Fig. 7.6c), the intrapleural pressure becomes positive ($+12{\cdot}0$ cm H_2O) and this summates with the elastic recoil pressure of the lung ($+5{\cdot}0$ cm H_2O) to make alveolar pressure equal ($+17{\cdot}0$ cm H_2O). A pressure gradient is again set up from the alveoli to the mouth. The diagram (Fig. 7.6c) shows that at one point along the airways the pressure inside the airway equals the intrapleural pressure outside the airway. This is known as the equal pressure point. The airways between this point and the thoracic inlet will be compressed because the pressures inside them are lower than the pressure outside in the pleural cavity. This phenomenon is called *dynamic compression* and affects mainly the larger airways. Once dynamic compression has occurred, the flow rate of air from the alveoli cannot be increased by greater expiratory effort. The higher the pleural pressure becomes as a result of increased muscular effort, the greater the extent of the dynamic compression, such that the net result is no change in flow rate. The only factors on which flow rate depends once dynamic compression has occurred are the elastic recoil pressure of the lung and the resistance of the airways between the alveoli and the equal pressure point. This part of the airways is known as the *upstream segment*; a confusing term at first when one thinks of it as describing the most distal air passages, but logical when one is considering the forced expiratory manoeuvre shown in Fig. 7.6c. In practice, flow limitation occurs in normal subjects when approximately one third of the vital capacity has been expired. This means that the flow rates recorded in the remaining part of the expiration will depend upon the elastic recoil pressure of the lung and the resistance of the small "upstream" airways only, and not on voluntary effort. This is where the flow volume curves are found to be most useful. (For good discussion see Pride, 1971.)

Flow volume curves

The flow volume curve is a graphic plot of flow rates achieved during inspiration or expiration, usually using maximum effort, against the relevant lung volumes. The flow is measured by a pneumotachograph and the volume can be measured by linking a spirometer into the system beyond the pneumotachograph or by integrating the flow signal to obtain a volume measurement. An X–Y recorder or an oscilloscope can be used to obtain a display (Fig. 7.7). The highest flow rates are obtained during the first part of expiration and these are effort-dependent. After approximately one third of the vital capacity has been exhaled, the flow volume curve peaks and proceeds down towards residual volume. The linear part of the curve after the peak is

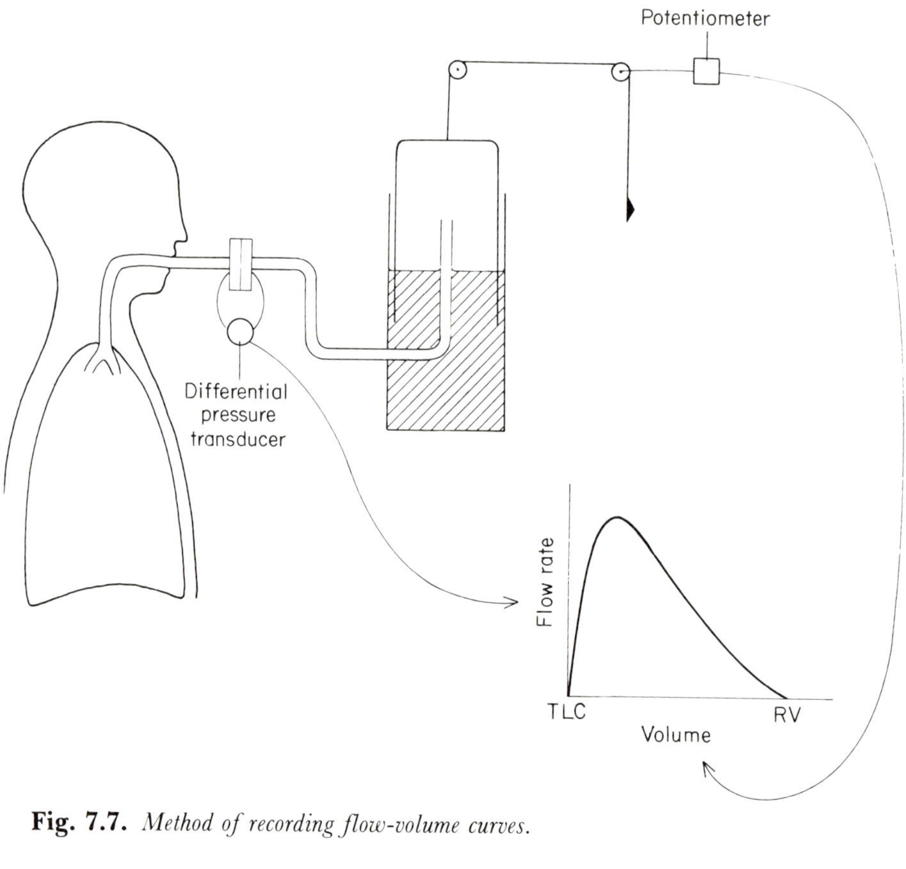

Fig. 7.7. *Method of recording flow-volume curves.*

called the effort-independent part of the curve. Figure 7.8a shows a "family" of flow volume curves generated by using varying degrees of effort. It can be seen that in those curves where moderate expiratory effort has been used, the curve joins the effort independent section at some stage. All sections, however, of the inspiratory curve are effort-dependent. One advantage of the flow volume curve is that an uncooperative subject can be connected to the machine and simply asked to breathe in and out with some coughing manoeuvres interspersed and the outline of the flow volume curve will be described by the line produced.

Figure 7.8b shows the typical changes which can occur in a patient

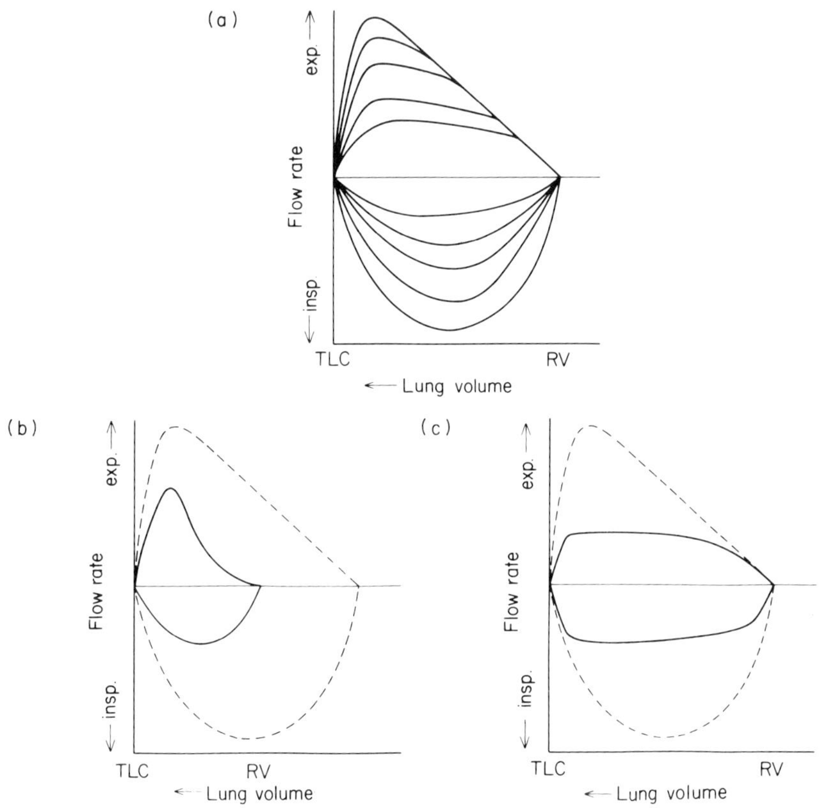

Fig. 7.8. *(a) Flow-volume curves in a normal subject using varying degrees of effort. (b) Abnormal flow-volume curve in airway obstruction (normal; dotted line). (c) Abnormal flow-volume curve in patient with upper airway obstruction (normal; dotted line.)*

who has airway narrowing. There is a reduction in the peak flow rate but the most characteristic feature is the curvilinear shape of the expiratory curve in the latter two thirds of the vital capacity. This pattern is often seen in patients in whom other lung function tests may be normal or near to normal. Also, the vital capacity is reduced and the residual volume is increased which are typical findings in the presence of diffuse airway narrowing (see Chapter 4).

Figure 7.8c shows a typical curve obtained in a patient with tracheal or laryngeal stenosis. The shape is quite characteristic with more or less equal restriction of both inspiratory and expiratory flow rates and with a severe reduction in peak flow rate.

Because each person's flow-volume curve is different and also because disease or drugs may produce changes in the size and shape of the curve, it is extremely difficult to compare flow volume curves between individuals, or even within the same individual between occasions. Any form of comparison of flow volume curves is difficult, although various techniques have been proposed such as measuring the flow rates at 50% and 75% of vital capacity. Measurements from flow volume curves cannot be routinely recommended for use in lung function laboratories, but observation of their shape may give extremely useful information with regard to identifying the cause of airway obstruction and detecting early changes.

Provocation testing

A characteristic feature of patients with asthma is that they respond to the inhalation of small amounts of irritant substances by developing a greater degree of airway narrowing than normal people. This phenomenon is called *bronchial hyper-reactivity*. There has been much discussion in recent years as to the value of this increased responsiveness as a diagnostic test for asthma. In patients with asthma, airway narrowing may also be precipitated by exercise, or by inhalation of specific antigens to which they are sensitive (Haydu *et al.*, 1974). These forms of provocation may be used in specific circumstances, but they are generally the province of the specialist physician who is trained in the techniques and aware of the dangers.

With non-specific challenge tests, small amounts of irritants such as citric acid, or sulphur dioxide, or of drugs, such as histamine (Cockcroft *et al.*, 1977), or methacholine, are administered to the patient by inhalation and the changes in lung function are recorded by spirometry or plethysmography. It is *not* appropriate to perform such tests on patients who have airway narrowing at the time of the test. In this situation, the response cannot be compared with normal because the base line is quite different. When airway narrowing is present, the correct test is to measure the response to inhalation of a bronchodilator.

Exercise challenge (see below) is safer for most asthmatics than the use of irritants and is frequently used in children. The subject has been extensively reviewed and described by Godfrey (1974).

Inhalation of specific antigens can be particularly dangerous in sensitive patients and it is not always possible to predict the correct dose to be used. It is advised that this procedure is not undertaken purely for the purposes of diagnosis, but limited to use as a research procedure for those who are aware of its dangers.

Assessment of disease in the small airways

The peripheral airways may be widely involved in disease, and yet pulmonary function tests may appear normal . These airways have been called the silent area of the lung. This is primarily because their contribution to total pulmonary flow resistance is only 10–20%, and even total obstruction of half of them would have only a relatively small impact on total airway resistance. A number of techniques have been developed to try to reveal changes in resistance in these airways (Cochrane *et al.*, 1974). One approach has been to see if breathing 80% helium–20% oxygen has any effect on flow rates found from the flow volume curve (Martin *et al.*, 1975). Normal subjects show marked increases in flow rates when breathing the low density helium–oxygen mixture. However, as flow in peripheral airways is laminar, and so not density dependent, patients with obstruction in these airways will show little improvement. Another approach has been to determine the point at which the small airways close during expiration. Diseased airways might be expected to close earlier (at higher lung volumes) than normal. This can be measured using a modification of the single breath nitrogen test, but the results are variable and not all authorities accept this test as useful.

When the small airways are diseased, dynamic compliance becomes dependent on the frequency of breathing. Measurement of the fall in compliance which can occur with an increased respiratory rate is technically difficult and has not proved useful as a test for small airways disease (Mills *et al.*, 1963).

Exercise Testing

The majority of routine lung function tests involve measurements made while the patient is at rest, but we must not forget that one of the most common presenting symptoms in respiratory medicine is breathlessness on effort. Clearly a method of objectively assessing this symptom is required, particularly when one realises that the correlation between subjective assessment or the results of lung function tests performed at rest, and the objective measurement of physical working capacity is poor.

Some patients, in whom no physiological abnormality can be demonstrated by routine lung function tests, may have some emotional disorder as the basis of their symptoms. This may or may not be associated with some degree of organic disease. The demonstration of normal or nearly normal exercise tolerance is valuable in such cases and may indeed assist the patient towards a full recovery. Conversely, patients with pulmonary vascular disease may display similar symptoms to those with emotional dyspnoea and the exercise test will help to distinguish between these two groups.

Occasionally, exercise is used to induce a particular symptom, such as asthma or angina. More usually, however, it is used to assess physical performance. At the simplest level, the doctor may simply go for a walk with the patient along a corridor or up and down some stairs while carrying out a conversation. Observation of how well the patient can talk whilst simultaneously walking may give a crude indication as to the patient's exercise tolerance. A more objective refinement of this test is the 12-minute walk (McGavin *et al.*, 1976). In this test, the subject is asked to walk as far as possible but at his own speed for 12 minutes. The distance covered is then measured and the test is repeated after recovery, the second result being accepted. This test has been found to correlate moderately well with such things as vital capacity and is beginning to be applied as a simple assessment of exercise tolerance. Its eventual value remains to be defined.

More information is obtained when heart rate, ventilation and gas exchange are measured. Usually this requires a certain amount of equipment and well trained personnel. A number of tests are used, including the treadmill and the cycle ergometer. The latter is the most satisfactory for use in a laboratory and any level of exercise can be simulated. Heart rate can be measured from an electrocardiogram and appropriate analysers and gas meters enable us to measure ventilation and gas exchange. Blood gas tensions can be measured directly but this requires arterial cannulation. Bloodless techniques are available but capillary blood samples from a vasodilated earlobe are now found to be satisfactory. Cardiac output can also be measured using a rebreathing technique (Jones *et al.*, 1975).

Exercise may be performed either as an increasing work test or after establishing a steady state. The former is to be preferred and can provide much valuable information. Exercise testing is safe although certain routine precautions are taken, such as stopping if premature ventricular beats occur frequently or if evidence of ischaemia is seen on the electrocardiogram. Pulmonary oedema may be precipitated in patients who have pulmonary hypertension.

The performance and interpretation of exercise tests is a specialised matter beyond the scope of this book. The subject has been recently reviewed (Spiro, 1977) and local laboratories will be able to advise on their own particular techniques.

Testing lung function in children

The need for objective measurements of lung function in children is as great as in adult pulmonary medicine. There are, of course, special problems related to equipment and prediction of expected normal results. Any laboratory which regularly performs tests in children should have the manual by Polgar and Promadhat (1971) which gives all the necessary information.

References

Cochrane, G. M., Benatar, S. R., Davis, J., Collins, J. V. and Clark, T. J. H. (1974). Correlation between tests of small airway function. *Thorax* **29**, 172–178.

Cockroft, D. W., Killian, D. N., Mellor, J. J. A. and Hargreave, F. E. (1977). Bronchial reactivity to inhaled histamine: a method and clinical survey. *Clin. Allergy* **7**, 235–243.

Dubois, A. B., Botelho, S. Y. and Comroe, J. H. Jr. (1956). A new method for measuring airway resistance in man using a body plethysmograph: Values in normal subjects and in patients with respiratory disease. *J. Clin. Invest.* **35**, 327–335.

Godfrey, S. (1974). *Exercise Testing in Children*. Philadelphia and London: W. B. Saunders.

Haydu, S. P., Empey, D. W. and Hughes, D. T. D. (1974). Inhalation challenge tests in asthma: an assessment of spirometry, maximum expiratory flow rates and plethysmography in measuring the responses. *Clin. Allergy* **4**, 371–378.

Jones, N. L., Campbell, E. J. M., Edwards, R. H. T. and Robertson, D. G. (1975). *Clinical Exercise Testing*. Philadelphia and London: W. B. Saunders.

McGavin, C. R., Gupta, S. P. and McHardy, G. J. R. (1976). Twelve minute walking test for assessing disability in chronic bronchitis. *Br. Med. J.* **1**, 822–823.

Martin, R. R., Lindsay, D., Despas, P., Bruce, D., Leraux, M., Anthonisen, N. R. and Macklem, P. T. (1975). The early detection of airway obstruction. *Am. Rev. Resp. Dis.* **111**, 119–125.

Milic-Emili, J., Mead, J., Turner, J. M. and Glauser, M. (1964). Improved technique for estimating pleural pressure from oesophageal balloons. *J. Appl. Physiol.* **19**, 207.

Mills, R. J., Cumming, G. and Harris, P. (1963). Frequency dependence of compliance at different levels of respiration in normal adults. *J. Appl. Physiol.* **18**, 1061.

Naimark, A. and Cherniak, R. M. (1960). The compliance of the respiratory system and its components in health and obesity. *J. Appl. Physiol.* **15**, 377.

Polgar, G. and Promadhat, V. (1971). *Pulmonary Function Testing in Children: Techniques and Standards*. Philadelphia and London: W. B. Saunders.

Pride, N. B. (1971). Assessment of airflow obstruction. *Br. J. Dis. Chest* **65**, 135.

Spiro, S. G. (1977). Exercise testing in clinical medicine. *Br. J. Dis. Chest* **71**, 145–172.

-8- Obstructive airway disease

Among the most frequently encountered clinical problems in chest disease are the assessment and treatment of asthma, chronic obstructive bronchitis and emphysema. The general description "obstructive airway disease" is often applied to these three conditions. The differentiation between them may be clinically obvious, but lung function tests are essential for a full evaluation, and frequently help in diagnosis. Serial studies in individual patients give an objective assessment of their progress or deterioration, and may be a guide to therapy.

In asthma, there is variable obstruction of the airway due to constriction of the smooth muscle in the walls of the bronchi and bronchioles, swelling of the mucosal lining of the bronchi, and increased mucus secretion. Between attacks, the patient may be completely normal. Chronic obstructive bronchitis is characterised by excessive mucus secretion in the bronchi and, although the obstruction may be partially reversible, there is usually a fixed element to it so that the patient is never completely normal. Emphysema implies that there is enlargement of the air spaces distal to the terminal bronchioles, and that there is destruction of the alveolar walls. Narrowing, or even collapse, of the airway occurs, particularly during expiration, and the airway obstruction is largely irreversible in these patients.

The diseases

Asthma

Asthmatics can be classified as either *extrinsic* or *intrinsic*. Patients with extrinsic asthma are usually young adults or children. They have demonstrable allergies to various substances as shown by skin tests or inhalation challenge tests. There may be other associated allergic conditions present such as eczema, hay fever or conjunctivitis. Intrinsic asthmatics are usually older when the disease begins (e.g. over the age of 40 years) and there is seldom any demonstrable allergy.

Attacks of asthma may be precipitated by contact with an allergen or irritant substance, by a respiratory infection, or by psychological factors. Young asthmatics are usually asymptomatic between attacks but in older age groups, there may be constant breathlessness. Examination during an attack shows that the patient is dyspnoeic, but usually not cyanosed. The chest is hyperinflated and prominent inspiratory and expiratory wheezing may be heard with prolongation of the expiratory phase of respiration. The chest X-ray may show hyperinflation.

Chronic obstructive bronchitis

Unlike most asthmatics, patients with chronic obstructive bronchitis are not completely normal between attacks, as an element of bronchial obstruction persists. They often produce sputum all the year round, but this becomes purulent and increases in volume during acute exacerbations which tend to occur during the winter months. A commonly seen characteristic of advanced chronic bronchitics is their tendency to develop chronic respiratory failure and right sided cardiac failure. Both of these conditions are usually fairly well tolerated. Dyspnoea tends to increase progressively. Examination during an exacerbation typically shows that the patient is cyanosed and dyspnoeic. Widespread inspiratory and expiratory wheezing may be heard and the expiratory phase of respiration will be prolonged. There may also be peripheral oedema and elevation of the jugular venous pulse. This appearance has led to the use of the term "blue bloater" to describe these patients.

Emphysema

Emphysema may exist alone, or in association with chronic bronchitis. There is no evidence to show that emphysema is a stage in the progression of chronic obstructive bronchitis, or vice versa. It is a separate disease process of unknown aetiology, although cigarette smoking probably plays a part. A minority of cases can be shown to have a deficiency of an enzyme in the blood (α1-antitrypsin) but the vast majority of cases do not have this abnormality as an explanation of their disease. As in chronic obstructive bronchitis, there is increasing breathlessness over the years and chest infections make this worse. An important difference from chronic bronchitis, however, is that respiratory and cardiac failure do not occur until the pre-terminal phase is reached. The emphysematous patient appears to compensate well for his lung damage and maintains a normal oxygen saturation in his arterial blood by hyperventilation. In contrast to the chronic bronchitic, or "blue bloater", these patients are sometimes described as "pink puffers".

Examination shows that the patient is breathless, but hyperinflated. The apex beat is impalpable and the breath sounds are distant. A chest X-ray may show a low, flattened diaphragm, a small heart and enlarged pulmonary arteries. There may be localised bullae visible, while some areas will have smaller blood vessels supplying them and will appear more translucent.

Lung function changes

In all types of airway obstruction, the patient has more difficulty in breathing out than in breathing in. The increase of intrathoracic pressure which occurs during expiration tends to compress further the already narrowed airways (see Chapter 7). This is particularly important in emphysema. The narrowing of the bronchi and bronchioles leads to the trapping of air distal to the point of narrowing. This is reflected in measurements of the lung volumes and capacities. In all cases, the residual volume (RV) and functional residual capacity (FRC) are increased to above normal levels. Asthmatics have a nearly normal total lung capacity (TLC), except during an attack, but the RV/TLC ratio may be raised. Bronchitics often have a reduced TLC but the RV/TLC ratio is still high. In emphysematous patients, both TLC and RV/TLV ratio are raised. The TLC can be as high as 10 litres and the vital capacity (VC)—or forced vital capacity (FVC) depending on method of measurement (see Chapter 3)—may appear to be fairly well preserved as a result. In patients suffering from status asthmaticus, the FRC is considerably raised and its return to normal is closely correlated with clinical improvement. The forced expired volume in one second (FEV_1) may not improve until some time later. The VC is generally reduced during an attack in asthmatic patients. Patients with chronic obstructive bronchitis usually have the greatest reduction in VC (40%–75% of normal). Emphysematous patients often appear to have a relatively normal VC, particularly if they exhale gently to avoid collapse of the airways and minimise air trapping.

In most cases of airway obstruction, the FEV_1 is reduced proportionally more than the VC or FVC. Thus the FEV% ($FEV_1/FVC \times 100\%$) is usually below 70%, and is sometimes as low as 25%. In many patients, however, the vital capacity will also be reduced. In these patients, usually chronic bronchitics, the FEV% is apparently close to normal even though severe airway obstruction is present. These cases might be confused with restrictive lung disease unless the peak expiratory flow rate (PEFR) is measured by the Wright peak flow meter. This will be normal when there is no airway obstruction, but is always reduced during asthmatic attacks and in patients who have chronic obstructive bronchitis and emphysema (see examples below). Often the peak flow rate is a little higher than we might expect for the reduction in FEV_1 in patients with emphysema.

If a bronchodilator such as isoprenaline is administered by aerosol spray, and the FEV_1 measurement repeated after 5 minutes, there is often an improvement. An increase of more than 15% is significant. Asthmatics may improve by up to 50% and bronchitics by up to 25%. The PEFR and the vital capacity may also improve. There is no significant improvement after isoprenaline in patients with emphysema. Severe airway obstruction (when the FEV_1 is less than 1 litre or the peak flow rate less than 100 litres per minute) will not normally improve after isoprenaline regardless of aetiology. This is partly because the inspiratory flow rates are also reduced and are too low for effective inhalation of the drug, and partly a reflection of the severity of the disease. If the patient's condition improves and the FEV_1 rises above 1 litre, any reversible element in the bronchial obstruction may again become demonstrable. No patient should be declared to have "irreversible airway obstruction" purely on the basis of lack of responses to inhaled isoprenaline. It may be necessary to

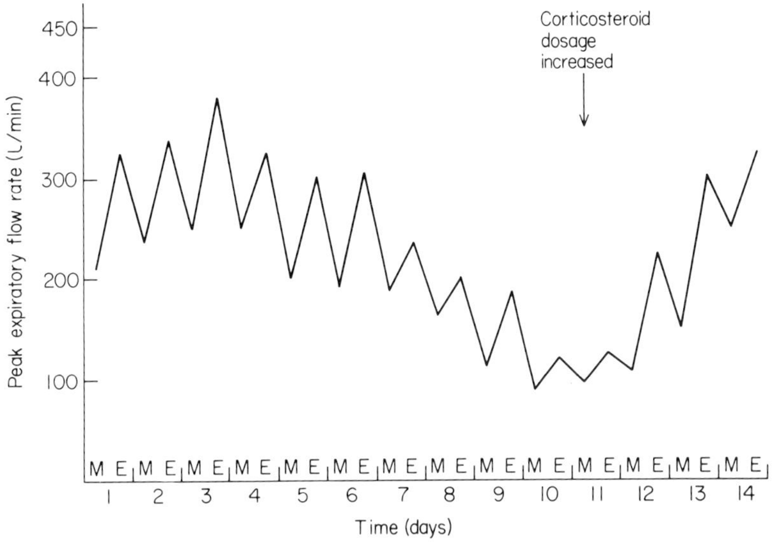

Fig. 8.1. *Serial peak flow record of asthmatic patient J. S. over a two-week period during which morning and evening values were recorded.*

give oral bronchodilators for several days to show reversibility, or in some cases a course of oral corticosteroids may produce a marked improvement.

Other methods of investigating airway obstruction are the use of flow-volume curves and the body plethysmograph (see Chapter 7). The apparatus involved is not usually suitable for routine clinical use.

A further feature of patients with asthma is their tendency to develop more marked narrowing of the airways during the night and in the early morning. This is sometimes called the "morning dip" and can be very profound leading to sudden death during the night. The cause of this phenomenon is not certain, but regular measurements of peak flow rate over 24 hours will reveal the typical pattern (Fig. 8.1).

The following examples illustrate the points mentioned in the above discussion.

Example 1

Mr V. C., age 48 years. Breathless for 4 years with wheezing. Diagnosed as intrinsic asthma.

	Actual	*Predicted*	*% of predicted*	*After isoprenaline*	*% Change*
FVC (ml)	2000	3000	66	2400	+20
FEV_1 (ml)	1060	2500	42	1500	+42
FEV%	53%			63%	
PEFR	120 l/min	460 l/min	26	180 l/min	+50

The vital capacity is nearly normal but the FEV_1 and hence the FEV% are much reduced. The peak expiratory flow rate is also reduced. After the isoprenaline has been given there is a dramatic improvement in FEV_1 and peak expiratory flow rate, and the FEV% becomes nearer to normal. These results suggest the diagnosis of asthma.

Example 2

Mr P. K., age 50 years. Has smoked more than 20 cigarettes per day for over 30 years. Complains of being breathless on effort.

	Actual	*Predicted*	*% of predicted*	*After isoprenaline*	*% Change*
FVC (ml)	1200	3000	40	1400	+16
FEV_1 (ml)	1000	2500	40	1150	+15
FEV%	83%			82%	
PEFR	120 l/min	460 l/min	26	135 l/min	+13

These results resemble case one, except that the vital capacity is much reduced as well as the FEV_1. This makes the FEV% appear normal at 83%. The airways obstruction is demonstrated by the reduction in the peak expiratory flow. All the results, including the small, but significant improvement after isoprenaline, are compatible with a diagnosis of chronic obstructive bronchitis.

Example 3

Miss J. E., age 24 years. Marked kyphosis since tuberculosis of the spine when she was a child.

	Actual	*Predicted*	*% of predicted*	*After isoprenaline*	*% Change*
FVC (ml)	1200	3000	40	1200	nil
FEV_1 (ml)	1000	2500	40	1000	nil
FEV%	83%			83%	
PEFR	380 l/min	460 l/min	83	380 l/min	nil

This patient's results resemble those of case two, except that the peak expiratory flow rate is normal. The reduction in the vital capacity is due to the restriction of respiratory movement imposed by the kyphosis, and the FEV_1 is reduced proportionally to this. Hence the FEV% is normal. The normal peak flow rate is evidence that no airway obstruction is present.

Transfer Factor

The transfer factor is usually normal in asthmatics. It may, however, be slightly reduced or at the lower end of the normal range in patients with chronic obstructive bronchitis and is consistently reduced in patients with emphysema. The amount of destruction of lung tissue by emphysema is well correlated with the degree of reduction in the transfer factor; hence this test may be of use in the differential diagnosis of airway obstruction.

Arterial Blood Gases

As mentioned earlier in this chapter, an important clinical difference between emphysema and chronic obstructive bronchitis is the occurrence of chronic respiratory failure in the latter. The "pink puffer" who has emphysema maintains his blood PO_2 until the end, and the PCO_2 rises only in the pre-terminal phase. The "blue bloater" who has chronic obstructive bronchitis will, at a relatively early stage, develop respiratory failure. Hence the PO_2 will be reduced and the PCO_2 will be greater than 50 mmHg.* These changes are exaggerated during exacerbations of bronchitis, but some chronic bronchitics are quite mobile whilst in chronic respiratory failure with PCO_2 levels of between 50 and 60 mmHg. In asthmatic patients, the blood gases are normal, or the PCO_2 may be low due to hyperventilation, except during an acute severe attack. Apart from being a diagnostic point, the measurement of arterial blood gas tensions is very important at all stages in the management of respiratory failure (see Chapter 5).

Summary

Although asthma, chronic obstructive bronchitis and emphysema share certain features, they may be distinguished by the clinical pic-

*For conversion to SI units see Appendix 1.

tures they present and by the differences in pulmonary function abnormalities. All three have some degree of reduction in VC and an increase in RV and RV/TLC ratio. The FEV_1, FEV% and peak flow rate are also reduced in all three diseases.

The most distinctive feature of asthma is a marked increase in the FEV_1 after a bronchodilator has been given, although absence of such a response does not rule out the disease. The transfer factor is normal

Table 8.1. *Pulmonary function abnormalities in asthma, bronchitis and emphysema*

	Asthma (during attack)	Chronic bronchitis	Emphysema
Vital capacity	50–70%	↓↓	Normal or ↓
Residual volume (RV) and functional residual capacity	↑	↑	↑↑
Total lung capacity (TLC)	Normal or ↑	↓	↑↑↑
RV/TLC	↑	↑	↑↑
FEV_1 before bronchodilator	↓	↓	↓
FEV_1 after brochodilator	Usually improved by 15–50%	Usually improved by 0–25%	No improvement
Peak flow rate	↓	↓↓	↓
Arterial $P\text{CO}_2$	Normal or ↓ (except in untreated severe attack)	↑ or ↑↑	Normal (except terminally)
Transfer factor	Normal	Normal or ↓	↓↓↓

and the blood gas levels are normal except in acute, severe asthma. Bronchitis is characterised by a variable response to a bronchodilator and a low normal transfer factor. The blood gas tensions are often abnormal and carbon dioxide retention may occur relatively early in the disease. Emphysematous patients have the largest total lung capacity of the three, and thus even though the RV/TLC ratio is high, the VC may be near to normal. They invariably have a reduced transfer factor, and there is no improvement in FEV_1 after administration of a bronchodilator.

Table 8.1 summarises the pulmonary function changes in asthma, bronchitis and emphysema. Some patients may not fall neatly into such rigid categories, however, and indeed clinically, functionally and pathologically it is possible for bronchitis to occur in association with asthma or with emphysema.

Further Reading

Fletcher, C., Peto, R., Tinber, C. and Speizer, F. E. (1976). *The Natural History of Chronic Bronchitis and Emphysema*. 1st Ed. Oxford: Oxford University Press.

Ogilvie, C. (1959). Patterns of disturbed lung function in patients with chronic obstructive vesicular emphysema. *Thorax* **14**, 113–116.

-9- Interstitial lung disease

The term interstitial lung disease is used to describe a number of conditions in which a diffuse fibrosis of the lung parenchyma occurs. Many agents can cause this (see Table 9.1) and in every case there is some degree of fibrosis of the alveoli. Often the pleura becomes partly fibrotic too, and indeed the whole lung "shrinks" leading to a restriction of lung volume. The fibrosis of the alveolar walls, together with a varying degree of obliteration of the pulmonary vascular bed leads to impairment of gas transfer. The characteristic findings in all of these

Table 9.1. *Causes of widespread lung fibrosis**

Cause	Example of resulting fibrosis
Infections	Chronic miliary tuberculosis
Chemicals	Paraquat lung, Bulsulphan lung, etc.
Neoplasms	Alveolar cell carcinoma, lymphangitis carcinomatosa
Occupational diseases	Asbestosis, silicosis
Collagen diseases and auto-immune states	Rheumatoid disease, systemic sclerosis, systemic lupus erythematosis (S.L.E.)
Extrinsic allergic alveolitis	Farmer's lung, bird fancier's lung
Unknown	Cryptogenic fibrosing alveolitis
Vasculitis	Wegener's granuloma
Vascular/metabolic	Left ventricular failure, "uraemic lung"
Chronic granuloma	Sarcoidosis

*This Table is far from exhaustive.

conditions are:

1. a uniform reduction in all lung volumes,
2. a much reduced transfer factor,
3. the absence of airways obstruction,
4. arterial desaturation, particularly on exercise.

In addition, patients with these conditions tend to breathe rapidly with a low tidal volume. This leads to an increased minute volume and in some cases, an actual increased alveolar ventilation, so that the PCO_2 may be lowered. The findings in a typical case are shown in Table 9.2.

Some of the individual conditions are now considered.

Fibrosing alveolitis

This is the preferred term for what, in the past, has been called Hamman-Rich syndrome, or chronic diffuse interstitial fibrosis. It may occur in association with a collagen disease or in a completely "idiopathic" form. In many cases, although there are no overt signs of collagen disease, one or more auto-antibodies may be found in the blood of such patients. Occasionally pulmonary fibrosis may precede signs of an illness, such as rheumatoid arthritis. Clinically the illness may present in acute or chronic form, the latter predominating. Chest X-rays of a patient with fibrosing alveolitis are shown in Fig. 9.1. In the acute form, symptoms of dyspnoea are present for three months or less and there are often constitutional effects, such as fever, tachycardia, malaise and weight loss. There may be quite severe impairment of lung function (Table 9.2), patients being cyanosed even at rest. Such cases are often helped by steroids, with not only subjective improvement, but a definite objective improvement in results of pulmonary function tests, especially with regard to the transfer factor (Benson and Hughes, 1972). Patients with more chronic disease are much less dyspnoeic and not usually cyanosed at rest, although they become so on exercise. They may run a slowly deteriorating course over many years and serial measurements of the transfer factor may show only a gradual decline. Steroids do not affect the course of this type of fibrosing alveolitis significantly. Both types may ultimately progress to death with right-sided heart failure and respiratory failure.

Table 9.2.* *Pulmonary function studies in a case of severe fibrosing alveolitis*
Mrs. L. J., aged 37

	Actual (ml)	Predicted values (ml)	Predicted (%)
1. *Lung volumes*			
Vital Capacity (VC)	2000	3300	61
Inspiratory Capacity (IC)	1200	2200	55
Expiratory Reserve Volume (ERV)	800	1100	73
Functional Residual Capacity (FRC)	1700	2600	65
Residual Volume (RV)	900	1500	60
Total Lung Capacity (TLC)	2900	4800	60
RV/TLC	31	32	—
2. *Indices of airway obstruction*†			
FEV_1	1800	2750	65
FEV_1/VC%	90	83	108
Peak Flow Rate (PFR)	440	410	107
3. *Transfer factor* (ml/mmHg/min)	12	28	43
4. *Ventilation*			
Tidal volume = 220 ml			
Resp. rate = 40 breaths/min			
Minute volume = 8.8 litres			
5. *Blood gases* (mmHg)	PO_2	PCO_2	pH
Rest	82	38	7.43
Exercise	54	40	7.39

*The lung volumes are spelt out in full in this table but abbreviations are used in Tables 9.3 and 9.4.

†The actual *volume* of the FEV_1 in cases of interstitial lung disease will be reduced in the same way as other *volumes*. The ratio FEV_1/VC will, however, be normal. This ratio together with the peak flow rate are taken as common indices of airway obstruction. This comment applies to the results illustrated in Tables 9.2, 9.3 and 9.4.

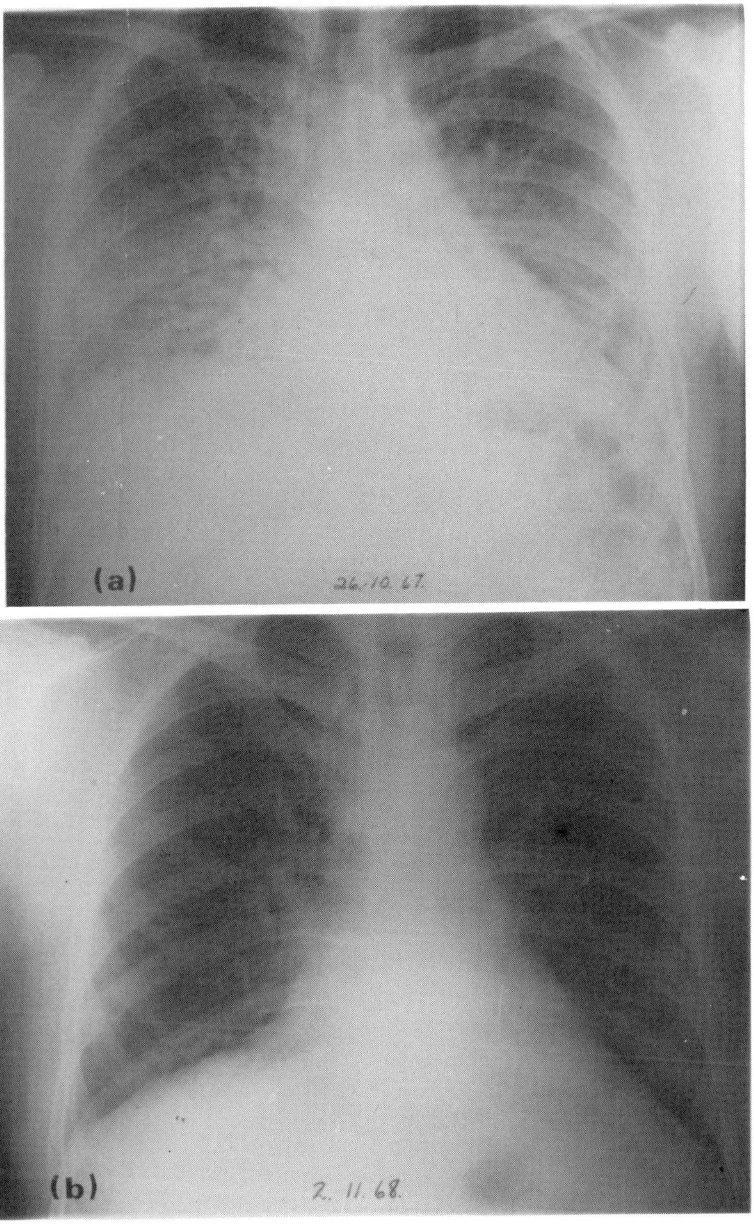

Fig. 9.1. *Chest X-rays of patient with acute cryptogenic fibosing alveolitis: (a) before and (b) after treatment with Prednisolone.*

In some cases there is a super-added infective and/or a "bronchitic" element so that there may be signs of functional airway obstruction as well. Serial lung function studies, particularly measurement of the transfer factor, can be useful in providing objective evidence of improvement with steroids or worsening as a result of the natural history of the disease. Presumably steroids help the acute cases by preventing organisation and fibrosis of the exudates present in the acute stage. It is perhaps not surprising then that they do not help the more chronic cases where fibrosis is already established.

Collagen diseases

The diseases most commonly associated with fibrosing alveolitis are systemic sclerosis, systemic lupus erythematosis (S.L.E.), rheumatoid arthritis and dermatomyositis, in that order. Polyarteritis nodosa presents with airway obstruction. In a group of 60 cases of systemic sclerosis studied at the London Hospital, 53 had a significant reduction of the transfer factor. Often, the lung volumes were relatively well preserved, as in the case illustrated in Table 9.3. Usually, patients whose fibrosing alveolitis is associated with collagen disease run a slowly downhill course and tend to die of some aspect of the disease *other than* the pulmonary one. Whether steroids help or not, again tends to depend on how acute the onset of disease is.

Sarcoidosis

A full description of this disease is outside the scope of this book and so a brief account only is offered. Sarcoidosis can affect the lungs in several ways:

1. bilateral hilar lymphadenopathy,
2. hilar adenopathy with pulmonary infiltration,
3. established pulmonary fibrosis.

Often these stages follow one another. Although some cases are first encountered with widespread nodular shadowing, many cases never progress beyond hilar adenopathy. Lung function is usually normal in stage 1 and often also in stage 2. The persistence of lung shadowing in

Table 9.3. *Pulmonary function studies in a case of systemic sclerosis (scleroderma)*
Mr. J. L., aged 56

	Actual (ml)	Predicted values (ml)	Predicted (%)
1. *Lung volumes*			
VC	3000	3900	77
IC	2100	2600	81
ERV	900	1300	69
FRC	2700	3300	82
RV	1800	2000	90
TLC	4800	5900	81
RV/TLC	38	34	112
2. *Indices of airway obstruction*			
FEV_1	2250	3100	73
FEV_1/VC	75	79	95
PFR	500	525	95
3. *Transfer factor* (ml/mmHg/min)	15	30	50
4. *Ventilation*	Tidal volume = 375 ml Resp. rate = breaths/min Minute volume = 9 litres		
5. *Blood gases*			
At rest	PO_2 = 79	PCO_2 = 37	pH = 7.41

the presence of symptoms of dyspnoea should lead to the suspicion that pulmonary fibrosis is occurring. Pulmonary function tests can be valuable in assessing the degree of functional impairment. If the transfer factor is found to be reduced (with some degree of restriction of lung volumes) this should be taken as an indication for steroid treatment which may reverse the radiological changes and improve the transfer factor. In a small proportion of cases, pulmonary sarcoidosis may present with a definite element of airway obstruction as well. An excellent account of the disease and its effects on lung function is to be found in Scadding (1967).

Asbestosis

This is considered as an example of industrial lung disease or pneumoconiosis. The pneumoconiosis panel in the U.K. will now take into consideration the results of lung function tests in assessing the degree of functional disability a patient has. The lung function findings (Table 9.4) are typical of any fibrosing alveolitis, although there are some features that are particular to asbestosis. The degree of

Table 9.4. *Pulmonary function studies in a patient with asbestosis*
Mr. J. F., aged 60

	Actual (ml)	Predicted values (ml)	Predicted (%)
1. *Lung volumes*			
VC	1800	3300	55
IC	1200	2200	55
ERV	600	1100	55
FRC	1900	2800	68
RV	1300	1700	76
TLC	3100	5000	62
RV/TLC	42	34	124
2. *Indices of airway obstruction*			
FEV_1	1500	2500	60
FEV_1/VC	83	76	109
PFR	450	480	94
3. *Transfer factor* (ml/mmHg/min)	12	28	43
4. *Ventilation*	Tidal volume = 400 ml Resp. rate =25 breaths/min Minute volume = 10 litres		
5. *Blood gases* At rest	$PO_2 = 78$	$PCO_2 = 35$	pH = 7.43

fibrosis is often greater in this than in other diseases with large masses of fibrous tissue being found in the lungs and pleura at post mortem. Radiologically the shadowing is most marked at the bases of the lungs and there may be a "shaggy" left border to the heart. Pulmonary function tests are of value in asbestosis and the pneumoconioses (Parkes, 1974):

1. to distinguish them from bronchitis;
2. to help to establish the diagnosis;
3. to assess the degree of disablement.

Extrinsic allergic alveolitis

This group of illnesses is attracting increasing interest and more allergens are continually being discovered (Pepys, 1969). These illnesses are thought to be brought about by a type 3 (Arthus) immune reaction occurring in the lungs. Precipitating antibody against appropriate antigen can be demonstrated in the serum, whilst inhalation tests (see Chapter 7) may be followed by a reaction six to eight hours later in which there is fever, tachycardia, basal crepitations and a reduction in transfer factor. Removal from the source of antigen may lead to a complete recovery as illustrated in Table 9.5.

Table 9.5. *Changes in pulmonary function in a case of extrinsic allergic alveolitis following removal* of the patient from the source of antigen*

	Predicted values	Measured values 2.5.66	24.10.66	23.4.67
VC (ml)	3000	1950	2200	2900
FEV_1 (ml)	2500	1475	1725	2150
TLC (ml)	4900	3925	4425	4600
Transfer factor (ml/mmHg/min)†	23	11·5	17·5	23·5

*Date of removal from antigen source = 3.5.66.
†For conversion to SI units see Appendix 1.

Intrinsic (cryptogenic) fibrosing alveolitis

The exact cause of this condition is unknown. Many cases have an auto-immune flavour, however, in that auto-antibodies may be demonstrated. Cases most commonly present with a relatively long history although some take a far more acute course. In some cases, there may even be an association with auto-immune illnesses other than those already mentioned under collagen diseases. One such possible example is the association with renal tubular acidosis.

Other conditions

Of the other conditions listed on Table 9.1, two more are worth a brief mention. In left ventricular failure, the lung volume and transfer factor may be reduced. Alveolar cell carcinoma is rare but may, like systemic sclerosis, be associated with a very low transfer factor in the presence of relatively normal lung volumes (Dyer, Hughes and Thompson, 1967).

References

Benson, M. K. and Hughes, D. T. D. (1972). Serial pulmonary function tests in fibrosing alveolitis. *Br. J. Dis. Chest* **66**, 33–38.

Dyer, N. H., Hughes, D. T. D. and Thompson, J. M. A. (1967). Bronchilar carcinoma: A case report with pulmonary function studies. *Thorax* **22**, 260–264.

Parkes, W. R. (1974). *Occupational Lung Diseases*. London. Butterworths.

Pepys, J. (1969). Hypersensitivity diseases of the lungs due to fungi and organic dusts. *Monographs in Allergy, No. 4.* Basel: Karger.

Scadding, J. G. (1967). *Sarcoidosis*. London: Eyre and Spottiswoode.

-10- Setting up a lung function laboratory

A lung function laboratory can be established with a relatively small capital outlay, but the returns in the form of useful clinical information can be considerable. Many hospitals and outpatient clinics already have simple equipment, such as peak flow meters or spirometers, but it is rare that the full potential of these items is realised outside a central laboratory. Although these machines can be used by relatively unskilled personnel, their use in a lung function laboratory by a trained technician with a clinician in overall charge will yield much more reliable results. It is only in this way that the equipment can be properly maintained and calibrated, and that patients who have difficulty with a test can be coaxed to achieve their best by an expert. In a central laboratory, the results obtained can be interpreted by an experienced physician and be reported and filed in an orderly manner. This means that comparisons over a period of time are meaningful, and that many difficult problems may be solved.

The minimum basic equipment for establishing a laboratory is a spirometer, a peak flow meter, and a Haldane apparatus with rebreathing bags for measuring mixed venous $P\text{CO}_2$. The spirometer may be of any type, but the simpler and more robust the better. A dry, bellows-type of spirometer (e.g. Vitalograph) is suitable. The Wright peak flow meter (Airmed) is portable and reliable. The Haldane apparatus is relatively simple to use, but care is needed to ensure that the potassium hydroxide does not spill into the mercury column or vice versa. The rebreathing bags should be sterilised after use (the usual central sterile supply department of any hospital group can cope with this). The mouth pieces and connections are kept in disinfectant in the laboratory. Oxygen cylinders are usually freely available in a hospital environment.

These basic items of equipment are adequate to make a start and to enable the clinician in charge of the laboratory to determine whether a patient has airway obstruction, how severe it is and whether it is reversible. It is also possible to diagnose restrictive lung disease and to detect carbon dioxide retention. In the vast majority of hospital patients referred for pulmonary function studies, this information is all that is needed. These items, together with a typewriter and a record system, can be housed in a relatively small room and could be purchased for less than £2,000.

A suggested layout for a results form is shown in Fig. 10.1. This type of form is useful as part of the report for the patient's notes and for the record system of the laboratory. The normal values for all tests should be predicted using nomograms (see Appendix 2) which allow for age, height and sex. The results can then be presented both as absolute values and as percentages of the predicted normal values. If

PULMONARY FUNCTION LABORATORY, The London Hospital, Whitechapel, London E1 1BB

Name:	Ward/Dept:	Hospital No:	
Age:	Sex:	Laboratory No:	
Diagnosis:	Height:	Date:	Consultant:

SPIROMETRY	Observed	Predicted	%	After bronchodil.
Vital Capacity (l)				
FEV_1 (l)				
FEV_1/FVC ratio (%)				
Peak flow ($l.min^{-1}$)				
LUNG VOLUMES (l) Vital Capacity Functional res. cap. Residual Volume Total Lung Capacity RV/TLC ratio (%)				
Transfer Factor ($mmol.min^{-1} kPa^{-1}$)				
Other tests:				
P_{CO_2} (kPa) (rebreathing method)		Normal range P_{CO_2} 4.7 to 6.5 kPa		

Comment:

Fig. 10.1 *Suggested layout for lung function laboratory results record.*

a bronchodilator is given, the new value, and the percentage change which follows can be easily seen. A report of the test should be written by the doctor in charge of the laboratory and the results and report should be recorded on a permanent index card for filing. A record should be sent to the referring doctor on the same day. As no complex calculations are involved, this should be relatively easy to achieve.

Once this type of laboratory is established, the purchase of further equipment can be considered. The next most useful item to obtain would probably be blood gas analysis apparatus. There are many different makes and models available and they are all expensive to buy and to maintain. It is advisable for any person who plans to purchase a particular model to consult with colleagues in hospitals where it is already in use to obtain their opinions of it, and also to discuss with them the suitability of the machine to the particular requirements of his own laboratory. Whatever system is chosen, it is essential that only one or two people are in charge of its use. The main problem with these machines is damage following their use by several different people with varying degrees of skill and concern. If an emergency service, day and night, is to be provided, staffing may prove to be a problem. A last important consideration when buying this type of equipment, is the availability and cost of servicing. A machine which cannot be fully maintained by a local agent should not be bought no matter what its other apparent advantages may be. Blood gas estimations are available in many hospitals nowadays as part of the routine chemical pathology service, and this may make it unnecessary for a lung function laboratory to have its own equipment.

The next most useful apparatus is equipment for the automatic measurement of the transfer factor for carbon monoxide. This type of machine is costly, and the test itself is open to some criticism, but it is valuable clinically in many circumstances and it can be particularly useful in following the progression or improvement of diseases such as scleroderma or sarcoidosis. There should always be facilities for measuring transfer factor in a regional laboratory, although the smaller hospital laboratory may be able to perform useful work without this type of apparatus.

A machine for measuring lung volumes by helium dilution is also useful, although it is by no means essential for routine work. Solutions for prick testing to determine the atopic status of patients are sometimes available in lung function laboratories, but in many hospitals other departments take the responsibility for this type of testing. Any additional equipment is more likely to be related to the research interests of the laboratory staff than to any service need. Examples of such equipment include body plethysmographs and pneumotachographs with spirometers and X–Y recorders for recording flow volume curves.

The laboratory should be supervised by a clinician who has an interest and specific training in pulmonary physiology. In this way, the reports will always have clinical relevance, and not become too related to pure physiology. Colleagues will only refer patients to the laboratory if the answers to problems of management can be provided in a reliable and understandable way.

The number of technicians required depends very much on the workload and in a small laboratory, a single technician may be able to perform the tests, maintain records and issue reports. More technicians, possibly with higher qualifications, will be required if any form of research work is to be undertaken in the laboratory. The training of laboratory technicians for work in pulmonary function is, unfortunately, not organised on a national basis in the United Kingdom although some local schemes are being arranged. In London, technicians can take O.N.C. and H.N.C. courses which include medical and physiological measurement. Some of the problems involved in running a lung function laboratory have been described by Hughes and Empey (1972).

Even today, there is a place for much greater development of lung function laboratories within general hospitals. The information obtained even with relatively simple equipment is of value to general and chest physicians, anaesthetists, and surgeons both in diagnosis and in assessment. For the small capital outlay required, the amount of clinically useful information which can be obtained by the lung function laboratory is greater than by that which can be obtained by any other department. Many examples of the value of such testing could be cited and a few are given below.

1. Pre-operative assessment before thoracic surgery

There is quite an extensive literature on this subject (Lockwood, 1973; Tisi, 1979), and tests of varying degrees of complexity can be employed. It is possible to predict from the degree of impairment whether patients with bronchial carcinoma, for example, would withstand resection of a lung or lobe. In most instances this can be done using simple tests—for example if the $P\text{CO}_2$ is elevated, this is a contradindication to *any* type of resection. At the other end of the scale, patients usually require a vital capacity of over 2.5 litres if they are to withstand a pneumonectomy.

2. Assessment prior to abdominal surgery

This is by no means always necessary. Performing simple tests in patients with a history of chest disease may identify those likely to run into trouble post-operatively. These include those with a very low vital capacity and/or a severe degree of airway obstruction. Such patients can then receive some pre-operative treatment and special attention in the post-operative period.

3. Pulmonary involvement in systemic disease

A good example of this would be the impairment of lung function in many patients with connective tissue disorders. Such involvement is well documented (e.g. Bates, Maclem and Christie, 1971).

4. Compensation cases

These have already been referred to in Chapter 9. Objective assessment by means of pulmonary function tests may be particularly useful in the pneumoconioses. In the case of asbestosis (Britton, Hughes and Wever, 1977), reduction of the transfer factor may be an important part of the acceptable evidence for the disease and may also be the first detectable change to occur.

5. Neurological and muscular disease

The respiratory muscles may be affected by illnesses affecting the nervous or general muscular systems. Examples of such conditions are poliomyelitis, infective polyneuritis, myasthenia gravis and dystrophia myotonica. It is possible to make objective measurements of improvement (or impairment) in myasthenia gravis, for example, by means of serial measurements of vital capacity or peak flow rate. Many other examples of these conditions could be given such as primary alveolar hypoventilation (Fishman *et al.*, 1966).

References

Bates, D. V., Macklem, P. T. and Christie, R. V. (1971). *Respiratory Function in Disease*. 2nd Ed. London: W. B. Saunders.

Britton, M. G., Hughes, D. T. D. and Wever, A. M. H. (1977). Serial pulmonary function tests in patients with asbestosis. *Thorax* **22**, 45–49.

Fishman, A. P., Goldring, R. M., and Turino, G. M. (1966). General alveolar hypoventilation: a syndrome of respiratory and cardiac failure in patients with normal lungs. *Q. J. Med.* **35**, 261–275.

Hughes, D. T. D. and Empey, D. W. (1972). Ten years experience in running a pulmonary function laboratory. *Br. med. J.* **4**, 470–473.

Lockwood, P. (1973). The principles of predicting the risks of post-thoractomy function-related complications in bronchial carcinoma. *Respiration* **30**, 329–344.

Tisi, G. M. (1979). Pre-operative evaluation of pulmonary function. *Am. Rev. resp. Dis.* **119**, 293–310.

-Appendices

Appendix 1. SI units

There is still some controversy about the most suitable units to use in pulmonary function measurements. Although a strong suggestion was made in Europe some years ago that the Système International (SI) should be adopted, there has been some resistance to this in the United Kingdom, and in North America, a change to SI units is not even contemplated.

For practical purposes, use of the SI system mainly affects measurements of blood gas tensions and of gas transfer. In this book we have decided to use conventional units. The appropriate conversion factors are:

(1) Blood gases

mmHg to kPa—multiply by 0·133

kPa to mmHg—multiply by 7·5

(2) Gas transfer

ml/mmHg/min to mmol min^{-1} kPa^{-1}—multiply by 0·335

mmol min^{-1} kPa^{-1} to ml/mmHg/min—multiply by 2·9

Appendix 2. Prediction and use of normal values for lung function parameters

From the nomograms illustrated in this Appendix, the predicted values of various parameters of lung function can be devised. The use of such predicted or "normal" values is not completely straightforward, however. Traditionally in clinical practice, the "normal range" is taken as being 80–120% of the predicted value. This has proved useful in the clinical situation although statistically it is certainly not valid. A purely statistical approach might be to regard values lying 2 standard deviations (SD) either side of the predicted value as being "normal". The co-incidence of the 80% predicted value with the 2 SD limit would only occasionally occur fortuitously. One possible approach is the use of the "per cent of the 'normalised' per cent of predicted" value as suggested by Sobol and Sobol (1979). This involves quite a complicated mathematical concept, however, and for practical purposes the use of the "per centage of predicted" value of the various parameters of lung function is likely to continue.

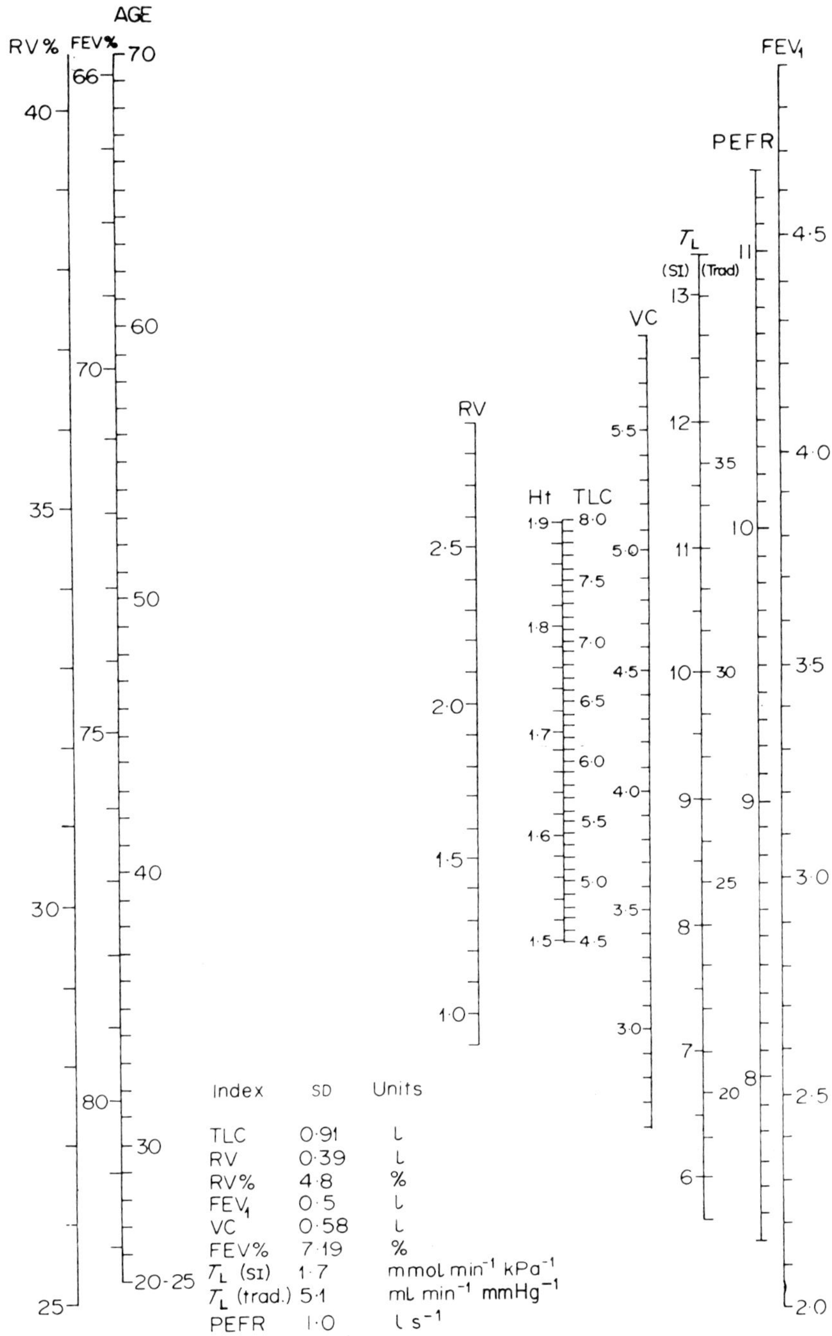

Index	SD	Units
TLC	0·91	L
RV	0·39	L
RV%	4·8	%
FEV_1	0·5	L
VC	0·58	L
FEV%	7·19	%
T_L (SI)	1·7	$mmol\ min^{-1}\ kPa^{-1}$
T_L (trad.)	5·1	$mL\ min^{-1}\ mmHg^{-1}$
PEFR	1·0	$l\ s^{-1}$

(a) *Nomogram relating indices of lung function to stature and age for healthy adult males of European descent. The RV% and the FEV% are related only to age, and the TLC only to stature. (Republished, with permission from Cotes, 1979.)*

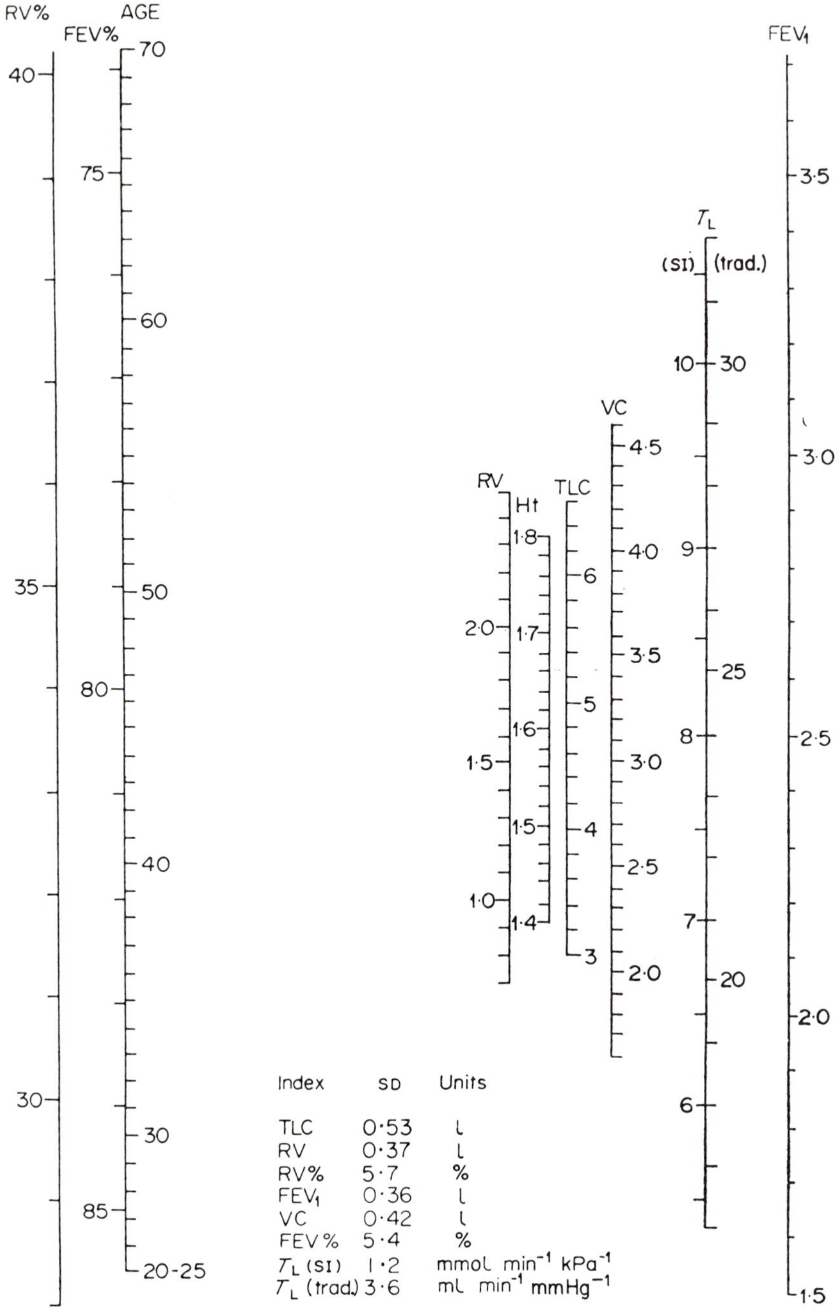

(b) *Nomogram relating indices of lung function to stature and age for healthy adult females of European descent. The RV% and the FEV% are related only to age. (Republished with permission, from Cotes, 1979.)*

Appendix 3. Symbols

Primary

D	Diffusing capacity
F	Fractional concentration
G	Conductance
K	Transfer coefficient
P	Pressure or partial pressure
Q	Volume of blood
$\dot{Q}$	Volume of blood per unit of time
R	Resistance
S	Specific conductance
T	Transfer factor
V	Volume of gas
$\dot{V}$	Volume of gas per unit of time

Secondary symbols for gas phase

A	Alveolar
APP	Apparatus
aw	Airway
D	Dead space
E	Expired
F	Final
I	Inspired
L	Lung
S	Spirometer
T	Tidal
tg	Thoracic gas

Secondary symbols for blood phase

a	Arterial
c	Capillary
$\bar{v}$	Mixed venous

Examples

O_2 partial pressure in arterial blood = P_aO_2.

Fractional concentration of carbon monoxide in expired gas = F_ECO.

CO_2 partial pressure in mixed venous blood = $P_{\bar{v}}CO_2$

Appendix 4. Standardisation of volumes

If gas volumes are recorded at the temperature and pressure within the spirometer then the values obtained are said to be at ATP (ambient temperature and pressure) or at ATPS (if saturated with water vapour).

These will need to be corrected to "standard" conditions to enable comparisons to be made. Two standards are commonly employed.

1. STPD—standard temperature and pressure, dry (i.e. 0°C and 760 mmHg, dry)
2. BTPS—body temperature and pressure, saturated with water vapour (i.e. 37°C and 760 mmHg, water saturated).

Since gas collection is usually made at temperatures *between* 0°C and 37°C the STPD correction will always involve correcting by a factor of less than 1.0 whilst the BTPS correction factor will exceed 1.0. An abbreviated table giving correction factors for temperatures between 15°C and 30°C (conditions in most laboratories) is shown below.

Correction factors for correcting gas volumes measured at ATPS to values at STPD and BTPS respectively

Atmospheric temperature (° C)	Correction factor for conversion	
	ATP → STPD	ATPS → BTPS
15	0·932	1·128
16	0·928	1·123
17	0·924	1·118
18	0·920	1·113
19	0·916	1·108
20	0·911	1·102
21	0·906	1·096
22	0·902	1·091
23	0·897	1·085
24	0·893	1·080
25	0·888	1·075
26	0·883	1·069
27	0·878	1·063
28	0·874	1·057
29	0·869	1·051
30	0·864	1·045

References

Cotes, J. E. (1979). *Lung Function Assessment and Application in medicine.* 4th Ed. London: Blackwell Scientific Publications.

Sobol, B. J. and Sobol, P. G. (1979). Per cent of predicted as the limit of normal in pulmonary function testing: a statistically valid approach. *Thorax* **34**, 1–3.

Index